MW00414423

YOUR

CREATOR

MATRIX

CATHLEEN BEERKENS

ILLUSTRATED BY DEBORAH CAIOLA

YOUR CREATOR MATRIX

How to Use Optimal Wellness and Quantum Healing
to Master Your Story and Create Your Reality

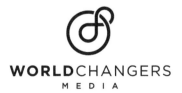

WORLDCHANGERS
MEDIA

Hardcover: 978-1-955811-63-7
E-book: 978-1-955811-64-4
LCCN: 2024900900
First hardcover edition: March 2024

Cover and interior artwork: Deborah Caiola / www.deborahcaiola.com
Author photos: Robin Caiola / www.robincaiola.com
Layout and typesetting: Bryna Haynes

Published by WorldChangers Media
PO Box 83, Foster, RI 02825
www.WorldChangers.Media

This book is dedicated to Source and Humanity.

I honor the resilient human spirit that has courageously navigated its way through the ages, playing out many stories of duality. With unwavering hearts, we all now step into the uncharted realm of a New Earth, co-creating our shared future destiny.

May these pages resonate with the echoes of your journey, inspiring courage, growth, and a collective pursuit of a brighter, harmonious, more loving future. May you be inspired to embrace your true power as divine co-Creators, evolving into the best versions of yourselves.

Praise

"Never before have we seen a perspective on manifestation like this. Through science and story, Cathleen shows us how we can create, refine, and design our reality by optimizing our well-being at the cellular level. This book will forever change the way you see yourself as an integrated being and Creator."

— **Marci Shimoff, #1** *New York Times* **best-selling author of** *Happy for No Reason* **and** *Chicken Soup for the Woman's Soul*

"You can feel the wealth of experience bouncing off the pages. This is a real story from Cathleen Beerkens of a life lived to bring us the foremost wisdom in health. With flavors of manifestation, epigenetics, and of course the importance of energy, this book will lead you to where we all wish to go A new earth and the future of medicine."

— **Paul Congdon, Publisher and Owner, Positive Live Magazine**

"This book is a tremendous treatise on becoming your best self. Cathleen masterfully introduces and expertly explains the emerging new sciences, most importantly the less well-known field of nutrition glycoscience, and how sugar structures build our cellular foundation that allow our body to communicate the metabolic functions necessary to create physical, emotional, and ultimately spiritual wholeness in our eternal journey to acquire more truth and light. This book will occupy a special place in my library."

— **Larry Law, scientist and author of** *There's an Elephant in the Room: Exposing Hidden Truths in the Science of Health*

"Cathleen Beerkens' *The Creator Matrix* is a visionary guide, seamlessly merging profound insights with practical wisdom. Discover the art of crafting and enhancing your reality within its pages while prioritizing your well-being. Cathleen's experience creates a roadmap for a fulfilling life where the power to shape your existence and nurture your well-being is firmly in your hands. An enlightening journey into the heart of personal empowerment. Just as Cathleen writes, 'Via your Creator Matrix, every part of who you are has a role to play in your evolution.'"

— **Maryam Morrison,** *The Eden Magazine*

Table of Contents

Introduction

Through my family lineage, I inherited a penchant for rebellion and change.

My father's Irish and Italian ancestors left the "old country" in search of a new world with greater freedoms and more opportunities. My mother's family was also European and were among the early settlers in America. This taste for change and adventure carried through to my parents and manifested as a desire to rebel against the status quo. Many of our family dinner conversations centered around making the world a more just and peaceful place.

We are all influenced by our genetics, as well as certain defining moments in our lives. Although I was shaped and molded by many positive experiences, those that had the greatest impact on my storylines were the ones that triggered my innermost fears. They sparked a journey of discovery that inspired me to search for answers about life's deeper meaning. This lifelong pursuit guided me to greater consciousness and mastery of health and wellness. I strongly believed that I could not do what I was meant to do here on Earth if I was not optimally well and healed. I understood, over time, that I could overcome anything because I am the Creator of my reality.

My childhood was bumpy, and I can pinpoint several experiences that propelled me toward my journey of transformation.

When I was in second grade, there was a boy in my class who had leukemia. Looking back, I see that it wasn't a coincidence that we became friends. We were drawn to each other and spent many happy hours together, despite his pain. I witnessed his suffering with intense compassion, so much so that I couldn't focus on my schoolwork. Then, he died. I had known that he was sick, but his death came as a total shock to me, and it triggered deep fears of illness, suffering and death. I immediately felt connected to thoughts that I could not trust my body and that the idea of death made living life paralyzing. I already had a deep understanding that these emotions and fears resonated with many of the stories told by the Jewish members of my family. Watching my friend die at such a young age, combined with these family influences, shaped my attitudes and perceptions throughout the rest of my life.

Just a few years later, when I was in fifth grade, I had a teacher whom I really loved. Her caring nature spoke to me in ways that no other teacher had ever done. One day, she told the class that she wouldn't be in school tomorrow, but that we shouldn't be afraid. Those words still ring in my ears. She went home and committed suicide that evening. It was too much to comprehend. This story triggered my fears again.

During my adolescence, as I was swimming in the ocean with my siblings, a rip tide came in. Suddenly I found myself struggling. The waves were slamming over me, and I couldn't catch my breath. I was never a great swimmer, and panic took over. I called out for help. Luckily, my brother, Paul, who is an excellent swimmer, rescued me. I had by then inhaled much water and it took me a while to breathe normally again. This near-death experience was a direct confrontation with my fear of death and made it very clear and conscious. I will be forever grateful to Paul for reaching me in time!

These experiences reinforced the fears and stories I already carried around suffering and death. Something deep inside me—my survival instinct—got triggered again. For years, I kept my teacher's picture and continued to connect with her sadness. While people told me she was "better off" where she had gone, I didn't believe it.

Later, when my parents got divorced, I equated that loss in many ways to the deaths I'd experienced as a young child. Every movie and television show seemed to be about tragedy, illness, and death. Once, I was watching a movie about a child suffering from appendicitis, and I had such extreme empathy that I could feel actual pain in my own lower abdomen. It seemed my whole being was attuned to others' pain and suffering.

My third big defining moment was not about me, or any one individual, but rather about groups of people—in particular, the Black and Hispanic communities, and their struggles during the Civil Rights Movement in the 1960s and 1970s.

My mother and father worked tirelessly with organizations that helped fight for civil and equal rights for all people. My mother became a political activist. While our friends went off to tennis practice or music lessons, we went to protest rallies. When our family moved to Saginaw, Michigan, we chose a house in a mixed inner-city district, with the intention of demonstrating that black and white people could live together side by side. Our neighborhood was peaceful, and we were surrounded by families of many backgrounds. I learned the greatest respect and admiration for Reverend Martin Luther King, Jr. and his gospel of non-violent resistance. From our family's perspective, at least, his dream seemed possible.

Then, in the summer of 1967, our lives changed forever. The Saginaw Riots tore apart our community. Police surrounded a house near ours and began shooting at people (regardless of color) in the street outside our home. I remember hearing gunshots, and my mother hissing, "Get the other kids and hide under the bed!" I gathered my five siblings and we all huddled together, praying no stray bullets would come through the bedroom windows.

After it was over, many people from our integrated neighborhood marched on City Hall and blocked traffic with a sit-in. Neighbors were beaten up by police, and more than fifty people were arrested downtown. In the aftermath, we were forced to move for our own safety.

The fear of death and pain were already deeply embedded in me, but this time a new layer was indelibly marked on my soul: the will and determination of people willing to fight for their freedom.

Within a year of the Saginaw Riots, Dr. King had been assassinated, but his dream lives on. In our modern world, we see new layers of the old stories about racism and separateness being peeled back and beginning to heal. Today's discontent is the foundation and the groundswell for a revolution of another kind. People still feel that they are not free or safe, and the time has come for fundamental change.

I realized, even as a teenager, that moving away from our neighborhood did not solve any problems. However, rather than distance myself from trouble, I wanted to confront it head-on. A world filled with fear and insecurity did not feel like a "home" I wanted to live in. Thanks to my mother, I got that chance.

Despite our experiences in Saginaw, my mother's passion for change was not diminished. After leaving that city, we moved to Washington, D.C., where I went to high school. There, my mom became the East Coast organizer for the social revolutionary César Chávez. Born into a Mexican American farmworker family, Chávez witnessed firsthand how few rights and protections farm workers had in the Southwestern United States. In many ways, they were treated no better than slaves.

Chávez became a champion for human rights. He represented farmworkers who had historically been prevented from unionizing. Chávez followed the non-violent tradition of King and Gandhi before him, connecting people all across the country with the call to free his people. Agricultural workers were living in shacks with little food and no medical care; and they had no way to voice their grievances. Through marches, strikes, and boycotts Chávez forced employers to pay a living wage, give other benefits, and eventually agree to a bill of rights for workers. With others, he created the National Farm Workers Association (NFWA).

I remember the grape boycott of the late 1960s. Our family went without grapes and lettuce for about five years. In the end, participation and perseverance won out. As Chávez famously said in his 1984 speech in San Francisco, "Once social change begins, it cannot be reversed. You cannot uneducate the person who has learned to read. You cannot humiliate the person who feels pride. You cannot oppress the people who are not afraid anymore. We have seen the future, and the future is ours."[1]

Alongside Chávez stood Dolores Huerta, co-founder of the

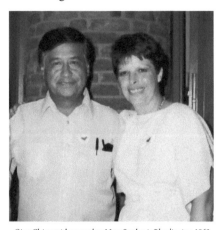

César Chávez with my mother, Mary Stephanie Blondis, circa 1968

National Farm Workers Association, and lead organizer of the grape strikes and subsequent settlement talks. The famous phrase "Sí, se puede (yes, we can)" originated with her. She was a strong woman who inspired countless other women to stand up for their rights. She also inspired me. I stood on the picket lines every weekend alongside the protesters working with Chávez, Huerta, and my mother, holding signs and raising my voice for change. Despite the huge job of raising six children, my mother still prioritized the struggle.

Through all of this, I wondered if I, too, could begin to make a difference in the world. If someone like Dolores Huerta—a woman from humble origins who, despite her incredible achievements, spent much of her life being treated like a second-class citizen by those in power—could lead a movement that gave millions of people the courage to create change for the better, then maybe I could too. I began to look around for what I could do to make a difference in the world.

Our home in Washington, D.C. was right next to the Walter Reed National Military Medical Center. Walter Reed is famous for being the hospital of choice for American presidents and congresspeople. It is massive, and constantly undergoing construction and refurbishments. After one major addition to the Medical Center, the neighboring families were invited to the opening as compensation for the prolonged inconvenience. My father wanted to go, and I felt a deep longing in my heart to go with him. He was always there for me and my siblings as a guiding force in finding our right career paths. From the moment we walked through the door of that hospital, I was struck as if by lightning. Strangely, it was as though my soul had found a way to give attention to my ongoing fears of illness, suffering, and death in a manner that could create positive results. I felt a tremendous pull in my heart to do this work, not only to heal others but to heal myself.

I had stumbled across my calling. Someday, I would work in a hospital.

Because of my genetic background and life experience, I was prepared to see this calling for what it was. I was excited to know my passion—an ideal that my father had been chasing from job to job and city to city for my whole young life.

Moreover, I felt that I had found my purpose for being born into this family at this time. Perhaps this *was* my reason for being here on Earth, and I had come here to this planet to help people heal.

It *felt* true. And so, I began.

From that moment on, I had an insatiable hunger to learn everything I could about human health. At that time, the best pathway for me was to become a registered nurse. It did occur to me to follow in my grandfather's and uncle's footsteps and become a doctor. However, there were two issues with this. First, I was the eldest of six children, and my parents still needed to put my five siblings through private education. I was not willing to take that much from them. Second, I felt a strong desire to help people through education, as I had already been practicing my whole life with my five siblings in the basements of our various homes. Looking back, being a nurse was far more difficult for me than being a doctor, mainly because I had to learn to truly listen to people and deal with their suffering up close and personal. Many of the psychics that I have visited along my path told me that I had been a doctor in several of my previous past lives and it was necessary for me in this lifetime to be in a nursing position. The twelve-year process in this role was definitely humbling, and I have tremendous respect for all nurses everywhere.

From my mother and grandparents, I knew that women's education was a source of prosperity and success for families and for societies. My great-great-grandmother was a suffragette. Isn't it interesting to realize that women did not get the right to vote until around the 1920s in many Western nations? In many ways, the work of women's emancipation still carries on today. I feel inspired by my great-great-grandmother and other courageous women who were willing to stand up for equal rights.

By taking this path to help others heal and emancipate themselves

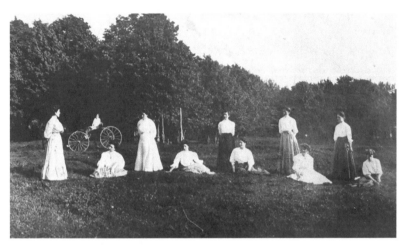

My great-great-grandmother, Alice Halpin Milard (far left), and her fellow suffragettes, circa 1900

from suffering, I felt like I was following in the footsteps of my predecessors, both male and female. I began my university experience studying psychology and biology, and ultimately chose human health and health education. I applied to nursing school at Georgetown University, where I came face-to-face with the reality of what was happening in our modern hospitals. After graduation, I worked in a surgical unit that specialized in ENT. I thought I would be taking care of people who had tonsillectomies; however, the reality was far grimmer. Most of the cases on this unit were radical neck surgeries due to cancer. It was the most shocking experience of my life. People were losing their ability to speak, eat, and breathe, and the surgeries were often completely disfiguring. I learned here about the power of the human spirit.

I started offering to give presentations for the nurses on pertinent educational topics, and eventually transferred to the high-risk labor and delivery unit, where I remained for many years. I taught childbirth education, worked with midwives, and began my appreciation for a more holistic view on health. Twelve years into my career, I moved to the Netherlands with my husband, raised three children, and eventually discovered my own healing abilities. My mother-in-law played a vital role in connecting me to my path of healing and became my biggest supporter.

After many experiences, some of which I will share in this book, I started to understand what connections are necessary to truly become healthy and well. I found many of the answers I was searching for through studying and researching the new sciences, and continued to ask questions and connect the dots of the complex underlying web of our changing reality.

In the Netherlands, I began to help people heal through the power of nutrition, emotional healing, energy healing, and spiritual integration. I specialized in reflexology, Polarity Healing, reconnective healing, and health and wellness coaching, among other modalities. The Netherlands was at the forefront of integrative medicine at that time. I began to spread the knowledge that I learned throughout the Netherlands and the United States about the complexities of health and wellness.

After many years, I was spiritually inspired to write a course. The first year of teaching this course left me humbled and grateful for the many hard lessons I needed to learn. I was a bit reluctant to continue, but that changed when I had a spiritual experience—at Disney World, of all places. I was with my family in the theme park when, suddenly, I heard a voice. (If this hadn't happened to me, I'd roll my eyes at this point in the story, too.) The voice said, "I am Michael."

I ignored the voice for the rest of the day. However, back at our lodgings, I realized that I was hearing the Archangel Michael. Upon this realization, I was humbled and began a conversation with him in the apartment. Michael asked me to look up Thomas and Michael. I immediately did so and discovered that he was referring to Thomas Aquinas. I already knew that Thomas Aquinas was responsible for much of the dogma of the Catholic Church, but I didn't realize that he was also known as the "Angelic Doctor." I realized that I had been communicating with Thomas Aquinas throughout the two years of writing my course, as I had been waking up frequently at night receiving metaphysical information about the connections between body, mind, and spirit.

At this point, I said to Michael, "I am afraid to continue with this course, as much of the information may not yet be accepted by the mainstream consensus."

Suddenly, I felt his presence come over me—and from that moment on, I no longer feared the rejection of the masses.

The biggest liberation we can experience as human beings is to free ourselves from our fears—in my case, the fears of sickness, limitation, and death. I was given the courage to put myself aside, take up the challenge, and totally commit to doing my part to help humankind awaken, heal, and transform.

An activist is defined as someone who actively campaigns for change. The world is in need of a huge shift like never before. It is not as simple as just letting go of our fears, but rather, about embracing the biggest change humanity has ever seen, a quantum leap in consciousness. Our Creator Matrix—the mind, body, and spirit complex that we will spend the entirety of this book exploring—is the vehicle for this change.

My ancestral lineage of creating social change ignites my motivation to bring this knowledge to humanity. This commitment guides me to create a revolution in the world of wellness. It is my mission to invite people to experience themselves as a Creator in their lives on all levels, and become their own individual forces for human evolution.

That's what this book is about.

How to Use This Book

If you have found your way to this book, it's likely that you are either seeking to overcome personal health challenges or to optimize your health and well-being for longevity, energy, and personal empowerment. This book will teach you to do all that and more.

Our health is directly tied to our personal power as a Creator of our lives. While many books offer information about how to use our minds and spiritual connections to manifest what we desire, my own journey has shown me that we cannot ignore the physical. Our bodies carry not only our organs and tissues, but also our stories, our beliefs, and our consciousness. Deep within our bodies lie mysteries about who we are and where we have come from. Our DNA itself holds information that goes far beyond what we know today. I am committed to keep searching for knowledge and am constantly amazed by the new information that shows up for me each day.

Ultimately, our body is connected to all aspects of ourselves, including the non-physical. It's *all* connected. In this book, you'll learn how body, mind, and spirit work together to create not only our current reality, but also our future possibilities. We'll explore the role of our personal stories, beliefs, and consciousness in our physical and mental health, as well as the power of the new sciences of epigenetics, nutrigenetics, glycoscience, frequency, neuroscience, quantum physics, neuroplasticity, bio-individuality, and more.

My primary goal is a lofty one: to contribute to the liberation of humanity by demystifying the process of freeing body, mind, and spirit from captivity. In this way, I am carrying on the work of my foremothers. By the time you turn the final page, it is my intention that you understand the power of your Creator Matrix—the web of information and energy that connects your body, mind, and spirit—and understand the significance of structure and how it affects function. Having this knowledge can help you find healing, set the foundation for quantum living, and ultimately become the best version of yourself—the version of yourself you were always meant to become.

I chose to call this book *Your Creator Matrix*. When I looked up the meaning of "matrix," I came across this definition, which spoke to me because it clarifies my intention for writing this book. According to vocabulary.com, a matrix is defined as "an environment or structure in which something originates or develops."

The word "matrix" has become very popular since the release of the eponymous movie, and many people have used it to define the out-dated, negative system we have all been living within. Although this may be true, I ask you to look at this word in a new way. Wherever we originate from and however we are currently operating, understanding the connections between our own body, mind, and spirit, and how those connections influence the energy and reality around us, will help us awaken to our full human potential. By understanding ourselves more deeply, especially the mystical role we can play by using more of our innate abilities, we become more of who we really are and deepen our connection to the Creator within.

On the following pages various people, ideas, and concepts will be explored. Many scientists, philosophers, and thought leaders (both contemporary and historical) will be introduced and discussed as they speak of this great change. Not one of them claims to have absolute truth or all the answers, but in their unique ways, these leaders are attempting to make sense of the new direction humanity seems to be taking.

Anything new requires change, and it is certainly apparent that with dramatic change there is chaos. As a child builds a sandcastle and then watches it crumble as the day passes, we have built systems and ways of thinking that are not intended to survive the next wave of change. The child on the beach has two choices of how to bring the castle back to life: smash it and begin anew, or try to fix what is broken. This metaphor mirrors humanity's challenges and how we will face all the change. As the old ways of thinking and being fall apart, we need to redefine who we are exactly and who we wish to become. The illusion that we are power-less victims of our entire human experience is crumbling. We are not the sand, nor the sandcastle. We are the Creators of the castle.

Vast numbers of people are awakening at this time. They are looking for new possibilities and ways of living. We are in the process of awakening to the idea that we are a Creator. We have the power to heal, manifest, and expand our consciousness like never before. By picking up this book, you have joined the fight for our evolution.

Welcome, Creator, to your bio-individual liberation.

Chapter One

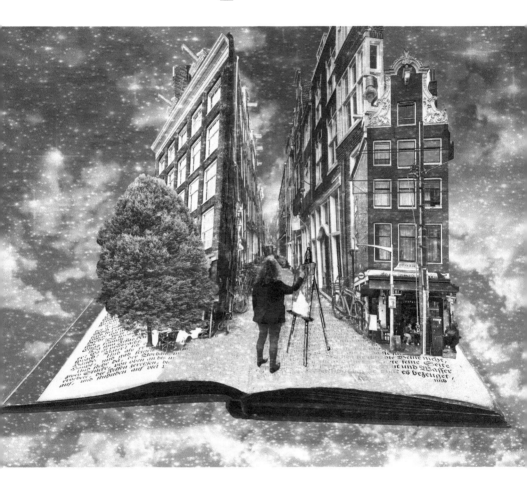

*How are you consciously
creating your story?*

"Understanding a question is half an answer."

\- **Socrates**

CHAPTER ONE

You Are a Creator

When I first moved to the Netherlands, my husband's land of origin, I was quite homesick. I suppose it is normal to miss family, friends, and familiar surroundings, but I had never been so far from my family before. Even for college, I stayed near home to be close to my family.

My first few months in the Netherlands were challenging. I only knew a few people, and everything was foreign: the food, the environment, the culture, and, of course, the language. Learning Dutch was a daunting prospect. It was hard for me to imagine feeling at home here.

After settling in, the discomfort was still strong enough that I felt called to visit a spiritual healer, who gave me a book titled *Hands of Light* by Barbara Brennan.

"This is just one method of healing," he told me. "One day, you will find your own way. And you will write your own book about it."

Still struggling to feel more at home in the Netherlands, I met a holistic Ayurvedic doctor, Dr. Levin, who had a tremendous impact on my life. She told me, "Your storyline is all up to you." She further explained that it was my choice how to proceed with my life from this point forward, and that how I chose to narrate my own story would greatly influence the timeline of events in my reality. Moreover, my focus and feelings about my story could lead to two possible scenarios. I could tell my story in a negative way: that I was forced to move to the Netherlands because that's where my husband is from; that being so far from friends and family made me lonely and depressed; that the people here were unkind; that the language was impossible; and that I had a horrible life. Or I could tell my story in a positive way: that I chose to come to the Netherlands to have exciting new experiences, and that, despite the inconveniences, this change could open doors to expanded awareness and opportunities I had never imagined.

Reflecting on the two options she shared, I realized that, in the first story, my dialogue was coming from a state of powerlessness. If I continued in this way of thinking, I would indeed become the victim in this story. However, when I considered the possibility of expanded awareness and exciting new opportunities, I could feel my heart come alive. Somehow, this version of the story not only made me feel happier but also helped me to reclaim my power.

It would take several years and multiple experiences with myself, my family, and my kids for me to fully understand this concept. But those early experiences helped me to learn that I was the Creator of my life and the director of my story. I learned that my thoughts and feelings were powerful, and that, when I chose a more positive way of thinking, I was exercising my power to create a more positive and exciting life—and certainly a more "expanded" life filled with greater possibilities.

As a result of my changing perspective, I made a definitive choice not to fall into the victimhood trap. I even took it a step further and spent time each morning thinking about and feeling how grateful I was for the opportunity to be here, in this place, with my husband and his family, immersed in his culture, and how I wouldn't waste a moment of it. It was liberating to learn that I had the power to make transformational choices that would affect the outcome of my future.

From this realization of being powerful came the understanding of responsibility. I knew that, if I was to take up the challenge of creating a wonderful life for myself and my family, I needed to take care of myself, too. I wasn't at all good at self-care, although I was great at looking after others. This imbalance was no longer serving me. I had to become what I helped others to become for so many years: healed.

There were, in fact, extensive gifts for me in our move to the Netherlands. Coming back from a burnout (which I'll share about later in this book), my first step was finding rest. My two older kids also needed lots of attention, and their needs—which included external professional help—were depleting my reserves. I had been searching for answers to their needs and dilemmas before our move, and in the Netherlands, I found them. As it turned out, we had moved to a country that valued integrative health and whose health system included many helpful and proven non-medical therapies. As a nurse working in the mainstream system in the United States, these more holistic ideas were difficult to find at that time. As I rested, I learned, and we all healed.

At that time, I met a practitioner, Titia Licht, who would later become a spiritual guide and teacher to me. Working with her, I healed the traumas that were connected to my inner child. Without healing *all* aspects of ourselves, we are unable to step into our own true power and become a Creator in our own life. What I didn't know then, but learned through my healing, is that deep within each of us we have a "child version" of ourselves. This child version is the part of us that comes to Earth with complete vulnerability. This part of us is often scarred by traumas and feelings of separation/abandonment. These traumas are often the root causes that create blockages in our Creator Matrix. Although I briefly explore trauma in this book, I encourage any of you to work one-on-one with a professional to heal these deeper wounded aspects of ourselves. Some call this "shadow work," which I discuss a bit in Chapter Four. Traumas that occur during childhood (above referred to as the inner child) can be especially impactful due to our intense vulnerability as young children. These set the baseline, therefore, for many of the limitations of our creative abilities later in our lives. I had to first heal my inner child before I could help others heal theirs. By allowing myself time and space to heal, reflect, and grow, I was able to do what I loved: namely, to read, study, and research. During this time, I had a third child, and she was more generous in allowing me time to continue my healing journey.

When you allow space for yourself, surprising and exciting things start to happen in your life. Some people call these synchronicities. I call them our creations.

Once I started to have space for new things and had recovered my strength, a lot began to happen in my life. While the kids were asleep in the evenings, I would study. I also started listening to people talking about the evolution of humanity and a "new age" coming to the planet. I was more than curious. I studied Eastern religions and started chanting. I started waking up to new possibilities: to myself as a Creator, and to the beauty of the world and of human potential.

Eventually, I started helping people to heal holistically. Through learning the new healing modalities, I experienced a new "expansional" energy. The veil between heaven and Earth was thinning and a new energy began to filter onto Planet Earth. This energy continues to offer humanity a larger bandwidth of frequency and greater possibilities to awaken and create. Over the years, I added many new modalities to my nursing knowledge: reflexology, Polarity Healing, Reconnective Healing, nutritional health science, and others. My research led me to the new sciences of epigenetics, neuroscience, glycoscience, and quantum science. Understanding health and healing in this new way was simply magical. And all of it tied into our amazing power as humans to design and create our own reality.

At this point, it became clear that I was launching onto a new path. I had always felt a calling to do something in the field of education. Now that I had been given so much essential new knowledge, I wanted to give something back and spread these new insights around. So, I started lecturing all over the country, teaching classes that I'd developed myself, and hosted many other like-minded teachers from the United States to share their knowledge in these exciting new fields. The focus was on introducing the new sciences and viewing nutrition holistically. Eventually, this led to the development of my health and wellness coach training course and the founding of my company, A Wellness Revolution.

What I and the hundreds of people with whom I've worked over the years have awakened to knowing is that *we are a Creator*. Not in some abstract sense, but in a very real sense.

When you realize that you have choices—that you are not a victim of life, of what's happening around you, or even of your past—your whole frequency changes, your energy transforms, and you slide into the driver's seat of your life. You realize that you are creating with every choice, every thought, every action, every feeling.

And so, the question becomes, "What kind of Creator will I be?"

What Does it Mean to Be a Creator?

We are currently in an age of awakening and enlightenment. Moreover, we are on a natural course of evolution, and evolution requires change. Change can create energetic chaos. Energy then seeks resolution in order to find the next level of balance. Ultimately, this process helps us to grow; with each new state of being, we see and understand more of who we truly are.

People on Earth today are going through a tremendous transformation, the equal of which has never been seen in human history. There is an acceleration of consciousness empowering people to gain awareness of who they really are and why they are here. Through this evolutionary jump, we will see more, know more, and understand more about this earthly experience.

When I began "waking up" years ago, I remember becoming very conscious of the difficult journey we all agreed to take by coming here to experience life on Planet Earth. To this day, I feel gratitude for every soul who comes to this world—a world that is often disconnected, chaotic, and full of darkness. We are magnificent spiritual beings having a temporary physical experience, and we are heroes in our willingness to experience the illusion of separation.

We are waking up to the fact that much of our perception of reality has been an illusion. The old systems and structures are falling; as we say goodbye to the old, we are being asked to create anew. Victim consciousness is slowly fading as more and more people choose a path of co-creation with Universal Source.

Each of us has an innate power that can naturally connect us to Universal Source and the energy of Earth. All masters throughout time have understood how to make these connections to rejuvenate, guide, heal, rebalance, and love. The more we connect to "the field"— the quantum grid of energy in which we all exist—the more powerful, peaceful, and happy we will be.

Becoming a Creator is, in essence, the ability to connect to all aspects of ourselves—body, mind, emotions, and spirit—and consciously direct the symphony of our self toward what we desire and intend.

If that sounds complex, that's because it is. But also, it isn't.

Let me explain.

Universal Source energy—also known as Universal Mind, God/Goddess, The Absolute, The One, or Supreme/Prime Creator—is whole and conscious of itself. At some point, it began to transform into smaller versions of itself, continually dividing itself over and over. With each division, it became unique and individuated; little by little, each piece forgot its connection to the whole, instead becoming an individual avatar of The One.

We are these avatars: unique, powerful spiritual beings who are nevertheless part of, and one with, Universal Source. Our physical reality and human emotions create the illusion that we are separate, and that Universal Source is something separate from and outside of us.

It is time, now, to wake up to our true nature and origin. The process of *becoming*—of existing in and operating from the integrated space I call the Creator Matrix—requires the full participation of all parts of ourselves: body, mind, emotion, and spirit.

As mentioned above, the world at large is undergoing a massive shift in this timeline. What is a timeline, you ask? At every moment in our existence, we are consciously or unconsciously making choices, both individually and collectively. A timeline is like a road—a road of potentiality. Through our thoughts, emotions, words, and actions, we are constantly influencing and changing our future timelines. As Creators, this gives us much more power than we realize to influence our future realities. Old institutions, storylines, and assumptions— along with their associated ways of being—are crumbling. Many of us who are lifelong spiritual practitioners feel an intense longing for "home"—meaning, the place in the universe where we originated, which is not Earth. Our job is not to check out but to tune in; to recognize that we are here, now, with a purpose. Although we don't have all the answers, we are here in this time as Creators, and it is for us to co-design and bring forward the new collective reality. The quantum leap in consciousness that we are currently experiencing will bring us a quickening of information that will guide us and help us master our unique Creatorship within.

One of the most powerful tools in our awakening process is understanding and beginning to direct our personal Creator Matrix.

The Creator Matrix

The Creator Matrix is my name for the vast network of connections between our body, mind, emotions, and spirit. Each of us is connected to this web of existence that brings forth life and provides a set of conditions in which we can function to exist, experience, and develop. This matrix is an environment in which we have all originated from. It is the "motherboard" of our holistic self. When it is functioning optimally, we have the capacity to create our lives deliberately, on every level, in collaboration with Universal Source.

When we are operating from our Creator Matrix, our body is healthy, strong, grounded, and balanced; our mind is clear and calm; our emotions are accepted and allowed to flow; and our spiritual channels are open to receive the guidance, support, and creative energy available from Universal Source.

As our medical and healing systems have become more and more scientifically based, we have created a system that is reductionist in nature. The amount of research is so vast that it has become almost impossible for the scientific and medical community to keep up. Years ago, as a nurse and a new mother, I felt the system was not working cohesively. When I would visit specialists, they often knew a great deal about only one part of the body but lacked the overall knowledge to understand the problem from a holistic or "helicopter" view. Although specialists have their place, people seem to be making a shift toward seeking out more holistic approaches to healing.

To understand how the Creator Matrix functions, it is important to comprehend that body, mind, emotions, and spirit are not separate entities. They are inextricably connected by a vast network of energy and information flows. Each cell, organ, tissue, and system in our body plays a part in supporting our unique power as conscious Creators. Our mind perceives and catalogs messages and information not only from our five senses, our broader environment, and Universal Source, but also from the complex cellular and energetic networks within the body. The mind creates, replays, and can ultimately rewrite the story of who we are—as you may already know if you've studied quantum reality creation—but the data that underwrites the story itself is stored in and acted upon by the body. Your story isn't just in your mind; it's encoded into your cells and your very DNA. Yes, your (currently) three-dimensional human body is essential to claiming your power as a Creator of your life. All energy expressed by the mind and spirit is processed through and integrated by the body. In fact, our greatest power is revealed when we feel balanced and healthy in body, mind, emotions, and spirit, and when all four are primed to hold and flow an energy of unconditional love.

All too often, people on deep spiritual paths neglect, resent, or even abuse their bodies, reasoning that "concerns of the flesh" are merely distractions from or impediments to their journey of co-Creatorship with Universal Source. That couldn't be further from the truth. Completely ignoring your body's physical needs (including macronutrients, micronutrients, glycans, proteins, fats, and toxicity) will almost inevitably manifest disease and imbalance in the body. On the other hand, hypervigilance around the physical body can leave you feeling like you have lost contact with your creative, spiritual essence, and can contribute to repression and denial of emotional, mental, and spiritual truths.

Via your Creator Matrix, *every part of who you are* has a role to play in your evolution. If we manifest chaos within any dimension of body, mind, or spirit, we will struggle to maximize the true power and potential of our Creator Matrix, and instead "disconnect" those inner circuits. When those networks are supported by a healthy body, a clear and empowered mind, and a clear channel for spiritual connection, you will be able to evolve your personal reality quickly and with far greater ease. Stepping into your Creator Matrix means understanding and doing the work to gain access to these complex networks. It is important for all these networks to be connected, and the only person who can connect them is you.

The first step in this process is to understand *how* all these multiple networks are connected. In this book, we'll explore the various ways in which your inner networks create, monitor, and ultimately evolve your power as a Creator. We will explore and redefine key concepts like consciousness, bio-individuality, wellness, and creativity. I'll share how the "new sciences" can help you optimize your consciousness, physical health, and path of action in this world by fully claiming and owning your Creatorship. When you step into your true, sovereign power, you will become a new version of yourself who can live and manifest multidimensionally.

Creatorship Empowers Quantum Living

Many of us live in a state of complete disconnection from ourselves, others, and the world, and have not yet integrated the different aspects of ourselves. To live in this state is to live in survival mode. In such a state, we are constantly reacting to, and often intensifying, situations in our lives that are not in alignment with what we wish to manifest.

To live the life you truly want, you will need to do the hard work of releasing the fears, traumas, old belief systems, and unhelpful emotions that are literally stuck in your body and mind. This is a large part of what we will cover in this book. These elements clog up and interfere with the pathways of energy and information flow between all levels of your being. In short, they gunk up your Creator Matrix! Trying to create your dream life without clearing and integrating the pathways of your Creator Matrix is like trying to drive a car with half its parts disconnected from the rest.

Our bodies are beautifully designed to hold high levels of light. When our bodies or minds break down, we often feel bad or sick; this brings us into lower-frequency states like fear, guilt, shame, and despair. These states impede our ability to receive and hold light. As you'll learn later in this book, this isn't just "spiritual speak," but scientific reality.

When all the pathways of your Creator Matrix are functioning in a synchronized way, you can attune your body, mind, and spirit to the highest energies of light. Light is information, and information—when transmitted to all levels of your being via the Creator Matrix—is the "food" you need to create joy, contentment, purpose, and unconditional love. When you follow the pathways I will outline in this book and optimize the intelligent network of your Creator Matrix, you will experience true, multidimensional living—what I call Quantum Living.

Creatorship Requires Personal Responsibility

Stepping into your Creator Matrix is a process, but it begins with a decision to take full responsibility for *all* areas of your life: your stories, your consciousness, your physical health, your spiritual journey, and your actions.

Everything you need to become a Creator in your life is already within you. Your power over your reality is sovereign and immense. Your work isn't to find power or sustenance somewhere "out there," but to turn inward with love, and recognize that you *are* Universal Source. Your Creator Matrix is the network that both amplifies and distributes your power; therefore, your first and biggest responsibility as a Creator is to maintain the integrity of that network so you can manifest your intentions clearly, quickly, efficiently, and in alignment with your true vision.

Many people today are still unable to manifest in this way and often find themselves manifesting what they do not want in life. Until we take personal responsibility for everything that is unfolding at all levels of our being—body, mind, and spirit—and do the work to optimize our own Creator Matrix, we cannot effectively do the work of changing the world.

As the saying goes, "Tend first to your own garden."

As a Creator, you will face your fears and work through them, rather than getting stuck in them. You will revisit and rewrite the story of your life, and use even your most difficult stories to help you grow. You will realize, truly, that love is infinite, and no one is loved more than another by Universal Source. You will learn to listen to your inner voice, take control of your thoughts, be deliberate with your words and actions, and move from survival mode to conscious Creatorship.

I want to be clear: being a Creator in your life does *not* mean that you will have, or should strive to have, power over others. To be a Creator means to be in your own pure authority, authoring your destiny and taking full responsibility for all the stories, experiences, and outcomes you create and co-create.

At first, it may seem hard to believe that we are such powerful Creators—that we have the capacity to influence what unfolds in our lives. It may feel easier to see life as something we have no control over—something that happens to us. In this transformational process, each soul on Earth will be faced with a deep mirroring of their ability to love and esteem themselves. And, whether we embrace our Creator Matrix and our innate power or not, the truth remains: we create it all.

For me, being a Creator has required a great deal of courage to change the way I think, the way I handle my emotions, the way I relate to those around me, and the world at large. Over the last twenty years, it has been necessary for me to really practice being a Creator in my life. The biggest fear I had in trying to become a Creator was taking on so much responsibility. I noticed how safe and easy it was for me to stay small. The practice of living a more conscious life has guided me to a more heart-based and focused mindset. I have become more compassionate toward myself, everyone involved in my stories, and humanity as a whole.

If you are currently in a state of merely surviving, or if you've been on a spiritual expansion path that does not include caring for all aspects of yourself (your body, mind, and spirit), this book will show you the way back to your power. Your first and biggest responsibility, therefore, is to begin to *feel good*. When you clear the communication pathways of your Creator Matrix to allow information to flow freely between your body, mind, and spirit, many of the challenges you currently face will be alleviated.

The biggest challenge you may face along this path is learning to exist in, and create from, the present moment. Many people live in the past; they continue to mull over what has happened to them or use past experiences as reasoning for current behaviors. Others live in the future, "wanting" things to come into their lives, but never enjoying what they have already created. When we are in our true power, we live in the moment of now, which is the only place from which we can influence the quantum field to create our manifestations and future states of being. As you'll soon learn, science is showing us that it is not possible to influence the field if our conscious minds are in the past or future.

For too long, we have tried—and been taught to—influence physical reality solely with our conscious minds. With the amazing power of our Creator Matrix integrating our bodies, minds, and spirits, we can, through our thoughts and beliefs, manifest easily and quickly. Everything is frequency.

As we undertake this journey to learn to understand and integrate your Creator Matrix, as mentioned in the preface, you will be introduced to many scientific and quantum concepts which may be new to you. It can be difficult to change old ways of understanding the nature of your reality. One thing is clear, however, and that is that change is inevitable and is happening now very rapidly. This feels like chaos—and, indeed, with any dramatic change, there comes some confusion. We feel power-less against the waves of life. However, we always have two choices: cry over what has been broken and try to fix it, or begin anew.

This is always our challenge as humans while facing change. As the old ways of thinking and doing seem to be falling apart, we need to redefine exactly who we are and exactly who we wish to become, and build new structures on that foundation. The illusion that we are powerless against the tides of life is incorrect. However, we must make different choices to create better results.

As you read, I encourage you to remain open-minded and remember that, in the end, you are the Creator of your world. You do not need to agree with everything I am about to share, or even embrace it fully, to begin to work with it and reap its benefits. As with anything in your life, you get to decide what belongs. It is in this discernment that we begin to find our own path toward healing.

Every Creator is Unique

As we are all connected to one Universal Field, we are one.

However, we are each a unique expression of that one. And, as it turns out, in order to understand how we can become healed, whole, and well, it is important to look at what makes us different, as well as what makes us the same.

In our current Western medical system, many treatments and therapies are designed to treat all people in the same way. However, we are now realizing that this is far from accurate. Our uniqueness is multidimensional, and, at this time, there are no methods that can fully evaluate this. This took me a while to truly understand, and I only really learned this through my own healing journey. Many years ago, as I was recuperating from my postpartum burnout, I met an Ayurvedic doctor, Dr. Lonsdorf, who, through pulse diagnosis, was able to determine my specific and unique imbalances and guided me to heal them holistically. This healing process initiated my desire to study and learn about Eastern medicine and ancient modalities of healing.

Even the definition of "wellness" is unique to each person. When you think of wellness, what comes to mind? Feeling optimal? Being free to be who you are? Being free to live comfortably and abundantly? Having enough energy to live the life you came here to live? As each of us will answer the above questions differently, it seems clear that there cannot be a single definition of wellness.

This is the foundation of bio-individuality. Just as our DNA is unique, so too are our preferences, requirements, choices, and creations. Our relationships and how we handle adversity further illustrate our uniqueness. No two of us came here to Planet Earth for the same purpose and/or lessons. Our life stories and missions are not written only in our minds but also in our bodies and energy fields.

Humans are influenced by nature and nurture. Nature brings us in touch with our physical being, helping us rejuvenate and return to our natural resonance and vibration. In the past, on Earth, we needed each other for survival. We counted on different types of energies to protect the tribe, work together, and harvest food and any necessities needed for survival. The male energy, the "hunter," was more yang, courageous, and protective. The female energy, the "gatherer," was more yin, nurturing, and cooperative. This polarity has been necessary for our survival up until this point in our evolution. However, the transformation currently underway is bringing us out of these rigid, dualistic definitions of "male" and "female" energy.

We are entering into a new age of humanity, known as the Age of Aquarius. Because of our advancements in technology, many of us are no longer struggling in the same ways. As these advancements spread across geographies and societies, we are seeing a great deal of advancements that are making life on Earth easier and less dangerous for humans. As we move out of survival and into Creatorship, we can become whole both individually and collectively, embracing all of the energies within ourselves and unifying them. With this change in understanding, we will change, and our relationships will change. We will have less need for dependency in relationships because we will not need others' complementary energy to balance our own. Instead, we will become both self-reliant and more accepting of the differences between individuals. This will empower all humans to follow their own true path and discover their true power.

Templates for Bio-Individuality

If we want to take care of ourselves and clear the pathways that empower us to create our most amazing lives, we must first answer the most ancient of questions: "Who am I?"

To quote Socrates, "Understanding a question is half an answer." In order to understand the question of our identity, we need to look more closely at what makes us unique and be willing to observe those factors in a way that increases our ability to heal and optimize them.

The "templates" for our bio-individuality exist at all levels of the Creator Matrix. They include, but are not limited to:

- *Mental and emotional templates*, including our stories, thoughts, personalities, feelings, and ways of relating to one another.

- *Spiritual and energetic templates,* including our consciousness, connection to Universal Source, yin/yang balance, and ways of receiving guidance.

- *Physical templates*, including our physical DNA, blood type, microbiome, cells, body, and ways of movement.

Our journeys, like everything about us, are unique. When we decide to love ourselves enough to create true wellness, our whole life can change. In this book, we will be looking at all of these in depth to support you in claiming your power as a Creator.

The first step in this process is to know how powerful we are. We have the power to become the observer and focus on becoming the best version of ourselves. This process can be quite confrontational and may be difficult to get through without someone helping you observe yourself. I wrote this book to support you in this observation; this is also a large part of the work I do with teaching my student coaches and coaching my clients. As we learn to observe ourselves with acceptance and love, we claim our power of Creatorship.

To begin the process of observing ourselves, we first must look at the most fundamental piece of our identity: our story. In Chapter Two, we will do just that.

Chapter Summary

- We are currently in an age of awakening and enlightenment, on a natural course of evolution, with an acceleration of consciousness, which is empowering people to gain awareness of who they really are and why they are here.

- Each of us has an innate power within us that can naturally connect us to Universal Source and to the energy of the Earth.

- Becoming a Creator is the ability to connect to all aspects of ourselves—body, mind, emotions, and spirit—and consciously direct the symphony of our self toward what we desire and intend.

- The Creator Matrix is the vast network of connections between our body, mind, emotions, and spirit. When we are operating from our Creator Matrix, our body is healthy, strong, grounded, and balanced; our mind is calm and clear; our emotions are accepted and allowed to flow; and our spiritual channels are open to receive the guidance, support, and creative energy available from Universal Source.

- Stepping into your Creator Matrix means understanding and doing the work to gain access to the complex networks of your body, mind, emotions, and spirit, and to connect them.

- To live the life you truly want, you will need to do the hard work of releasing the fears, old traumas, old belief systems, and unhelpful emotions that are stuck in your body and mind, because these clog and impair your Creator Matrix.

- When all the pathways of your Creator Matrix are functioning in a synchronized way, you can attune your body, mind, emotions, and spirit to the highest energies of light. Light is information and the "food" you need to create joy, contentment, purpose, and unconditional love.

- This book will help you maintain the integrity and optimize the intelligent network of your Creator Matrix and experience true, multidimensional Quantum Living.

- To achieve this, we need to take full responsibility for all areas of our lives: our stories, our consciousness, our physical health, our spiritual journey, and our actions.

- We can only influence the quantum field in the moment of now to create our manifestations and future states of being.

- We are all connected to one Universal Field, so we are one. However, we are each a unique expression of that "one." The templates for our bio-individuality exist at all levels of our Creator Matrix.

- Our whole life can change when we decide to love ourselves enough to create true wellness.

- The first step to claiming our power as a Creator is to become the observer and focus on becoming the best version of ourselves.

Chapter Two

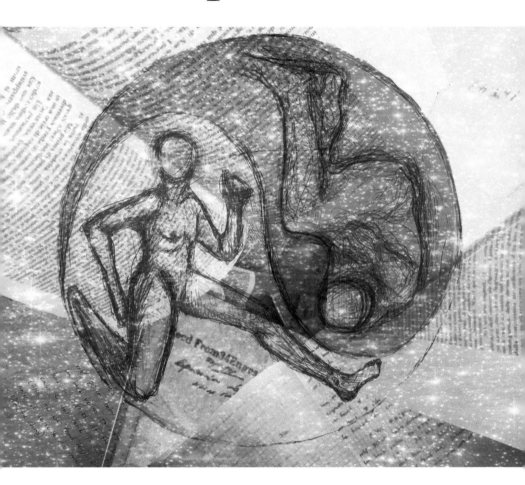

*How are you nourishing and
balancing your Creator Matrix to
manifest your desired reality?*

"The first step toward change is awareness.
The second step is acceptance."

- Nathaniel Branden

CHAPTER TWO

The Art of Manifestation and Digestion

I t would be wonderful if, when we were born, we received a manual to help us understand why we are here on Planet Earth and what we are here to do. It would be so helpful for us to understand the nature of this earthly reality and the complexities of maneuvering ourselves through it.

As it is, though, most of us learn about this interconnectedness through our own experiences and life stories. Unfortunately, many times, we learn the hard way. And, when we do become aware that we create our reality, most of us struggle with the process of bringing the life we desire into being, because we are not fully aware of the constant dance and interconnectedness between our inner world and what is showing up in our outer world.

My son, Frans Jr., was born on my birthday—which sounds great, but was, in fact, exhausting. He was overdue by two weeks, and I had been working non-stop at the hospital in a very tense maternity and natal care ward. I was very pregnant, swollen, switching between day and night shifts, and not listening to my body at all. Rather than sticking to the nutritious diet I was recommending to other pregnant women, I was getting through night shifts by wolfing down pizzas and gorging on sugary donuts, washed down with *lots* of coffee.

While many mothers work full-time right up until the moment of delivery and then go on to have easy births and healthy babies, that was not my story. My work was heavy and stressful, and included lifting people and assisting during complicated births (such as delivering quadruplets and babies with health challenges.) There were plenty of emotional shocks, daily emergencies, and mothers screaming in pain. Every birth has its own story, and its own suspense.

Looking back, I feel lucky I didn't lose my son.

After he was two weeks overdue, I was induced with the intention of having a vaginal birth. For twenty-four hours, we had tried everything, but his head was simply too big to pass through the birth canal. His heart rate started to drop, and I was wheeled off to have an emergency cesarean section because my son was in fetal distress.

That alone would have been stressful enough, but that was only the beginning. My adorable son, weighing in at nine pounds, three ounces, was not breathing well. So, they whisked him off to the NICU—where he was easily the largest baby on the ward.

My husband, Frans, was stressed and exhausted. I was stressed and exhausted. After stitching up my abdomen, they gave me morphine for the pain, not realizing that I have an allergy to morphine—so that made everything worse. I did not see my son until the next day, and it was then that his health challenges really began. He was given a lot of antibiotics, which probably saved his life, but they left him weak and sickly for two years.

As a nurse, I felt stigmatized for not having a healthy baby. When I went back to work full-time, we hired a caregiver for Frans Jr. whom we later found out was HIV-positive. Much less was known about HIV back then and there was a great deal of fear surrounding it. My son was still struggling with a compromised immune system. Thankfully we now know that HIV is not contracted in this way, but we didn't know that at the time. However, my fears had gotten the best of me, and I remained unsure about how to handle his chronic respiratory issues.

I had taken him to many doctors at Johns Hopkins with no clear solutions. I was desperate to find answers for him and felt disappointed in mainstream medicine.

A breakthrough occurred when we took my son for treatment with a cranio-osteopath. I had heard from a cousin in Europe how much her practitioner had helped her son. After one treatment with the practitioner I found in the US, he concluded that my son's cranium was not moving as it should. He explained that, when babies are born through the birth canal, their cranium is stimulated to move in a healthy way. My son never made it naturally through the birth canal; instead, his head was repeatedly pushed against my cervix, so his cranium was jammed, and this was having a debilitating effect on the health of his entire system, including his nervous system, digestive system, and immune system. It showed up physically as chronic immune infections, and mentally and emotionally as a severely irritable and overstimulated nervous system.

Week after week, I took Frans Jr. to this practitioner—and, to my surprise, his health began to improve. He was having fewer respiratory infections, his acute asthmatic episodes decreased, his chronic digestive discomfort subsided, and he seemed calmer and happier overall. Working with this practitioner was my first experience with integrative medicine and I was amazed that he was able to help my son heal so quickly. Within two months, he was off all of his medications, including his inhaler, and was sleeping much better.

When we moved to the Netherlands, our family got a lot of support from my mother-in-law on all levels. We lived with her at first; she helped us get settled and has been a tremendous support to us for all these years. At some point she recommended that I see her friend, a kinesiologist named José Vergroesen, as I was out of balance and experiencing anxiety as I adjusted to the new culture. This is where my healing journey began. It is amazing to me how interconnected we all are. If I hadn't gotten her referral, I might not have healed myself and my family and therefore would not be helping others like I do today. Healing is a complex process and all levels of existence (body, mind, and spirit) matter. I learned from José that healing is not as simple as just taking medicine or having one healing treatment. It is a journey, and like peeling an onion, it starts with an intention to heal on all levels. We are grateful for meeting José as she helped our family to heal.

At some point in the early years living in the Netherlands, I decided to take my son to her, as he was experiencing fears and bouts of eczema. As mentioned above, I had been helping my son heal his physical trauma from birth. However, I learned through José that my son had also suffered a sort of emotional trauma from the birth. He had been taken to intensive care immediately after delivery, instead of being placed in my arms, which was a shock to him. This caused emotional blockages that we worked on and resolved over the years. I also took my son to an orthomolecular therapist to help resolve his eczema. She found his diet was a cause of his weakened immune system contributing to the eczema. With her help we made dietary changes. We cut out all refined sugar except for once a week and added in organic supplements to support his healing. His whole system improved dramatically over the course of the subsequent year. These experiences reinforced the power of healing on all levels of body, mind, and spirit, and taught me that illness and trauma can occur on all these levels too.

I learned many lessons through my children in the subsequent ten years that helped me search for the underlying root cause of issues that compromised their, and my, optimal health. I learned not only how to treat the symptoms but also how to uncover the root causes of the imbalances. I was constantly amazed at how easy it was for my children to heal and rebalance. Because of these successes, I began to turn to these new healing modalities more regularly. Although supporting my son as an infant was my first experience with integrative medicine, it was just the beginning of my journey into the world of holistic healing—and what I learned would change my life and those around me forever.

The stories of my experiences created a framework for the direction my life would take. They also helped me see how I have impacted my stories through my choices, thoughts, and emotions. My stories impact me, but I also impact them.

Through my studies, I became aware of two key forces of creation that influence our power to bring what we desire into our reality, including our health. To become a powerful Creator, we must master both. The first force is manifestation, which gives us the power to influence our reality. The second is digestion, which gives us the power to integrate the effects of our experiences and stories upon us.

When we understand the creative cycle of manifestation and digestion, we can support our body-mind-spirit matrix. To successfully manifest what we desire, we must keep our matrix vital and clear, and visualize where we want to go as we begin a new creative cycle. We must also take the time to digest and integrate who we have become from our past life stories so we are ready for the next steps.

In this chapter, we will look at this cycle of manifestation and digestion and how these two forces of creation can support us in becoming the amazing Creators we are meant to be.

We Create Our Stories

Can you imagine what it would be like to feel amazing every day, full of energy, inspiration, appreciation, and love? Can you imagine what it would be like to feel fully alive and present in every moment? Can you imagine what it would be like to know that, through your Creator Matrix, you can successfully manifest anything and everything you want instantly?

That would be an amazing experience!

But if you're like most people, the moment you read the words above, you started telling yourself a story about why you *can't* have those things. Why you are different from those people who seem to manifest everything they desire. Why people who can easily manifest are luckier or smarter or more beloved of Universal Source than you are. Why you can live a life of joy and presence sometimes, but definitely not *all* the time.

Those questions, feelings, and fears are your stories making themselves known. We are here on Earth to learn to manifest, and eventually this will become self-evident.

The word "manifest" feels "New-Agey" to many people, but to me it is simply another word that describes our process as Creators. To manifest means to bring into physical form through intention in the energetic field. It has been described by many as "having your dreams come true," "making your vision a reality," and "bringing your story to life." For our purposes, we will define manifesting as "how our consciousness directly affects our reality."

When we begin to work within our Creator Matrix and explore full-spectrum wellness, our first point of attention must always be our stories, because our stories touch, influence, and shape everything about our multidimensional selves. Until we learn to identify, digest, and consciously shape our stories, we will not be able to create optimal well-being on all levels.

The process of working with your stories begins with self-reflection. What do you tell yourself about yourself, every day? How have your ways of living and the stories you tell yourself about your life decisions served your soul and your reason for being here on Earth? Once we begin to ask questions like these, we can invite new possibilities to arise.

In the past, many of us, myself included, were so busy surviving and coping with challenge after challenge that we did not have time to look at the stories we told ourselves about who we are, what we do, and why we are who we are. The first seven years of life are when we develop many of the beliefs, values, and habits that guide us throughout our lives. But during those years, were we taught how to be our best selves, and how to take care of the whole of ourselves—body, mind, and spirit? For most of us, the answer is "no." We simply did the best with the knowledge, perspectives, and experiences we were given, and built stories around these elements that eventually became the definition of "us."

As I mentioned earlier, while it would be nice to have been given a guidebook for navigating life on Planet Earth in a human body, few, if any, of us were given such a resource. Most of us need to wake up to the fact that we are Creators, and that, through our actions, reactions, responses, and beliefs, we make things happen in our lives. Our stories are the driving force behind all those things.

As I've shared, I come from a large family of six children, and we were busy with day-to-day family life. My parents were teachers (my dad a chemist), and, as mentioned in the introduction, they were both concerned with helping the community. Their love for others made a tremendous impression on all six of us. However, because the focus was on helping others, caring for ourselves and tending to our own needs was not on the radar. Until the birth of my son, I was still immersed in my story that serving others meant neglecting myself. My experience with his traumatic birth and difficult early years helped me see that that story was not serving me.

Looking back at all the years of raising my children, my biggest lesson by far was to learn to care for myself. As the eldest child, I was always busy helping my parents take care of my younger siblings. As I went on to college and subsequently became a teacher and nurse, this pattern of caring for others continued. By the time I delivered Frans Jr., I was out of balance, burned out, and experiencing postpartum depression. In addition to caring for him, I also needed to learn to care for myself. Working with patients, clients, and students over many years, I recognize that this seems to be an overall recurring theme for most of humanity.

By the time I had my other two children, I had learned to make better choices about my health that ensured that the depression did not recur. Again, because I had always focused on caring for others, it took this experience with my own child for me to fully understand and appreciate the SOS my body, mind, and spirit were sending me, and how my own wellness impacted my ability to create the life I wanted for both them and me.

When you fly on a plane, they tell you to always put on your own oxygen mask first. I learned this the hard way. My story about self-care, and what it meant to truly take care of myself, was influenced by my inner stories about my value in the world, which were in turn influenced by my experiences growing up.

Our body, mind, and spirit can all be injured by pain and sudden shocks to our system. When the shock appears to be confined to one level of our being, it can be easy to underestimate its significance. However, our Creator Matrix channels information at and through all levels of our being; this means that a physical shock can create energetic blockages at the mental and spiritual levels as well. We saw this with my son: the traumatic birth affected him physically, but also emotionally—and that emotional impact showed up years later as physical symptoms! When these blocks are not dealt with in a timely manner, but rather integrated into our ongoing inner narratives about who we are and what is (and is not) possible for us, they can eventually cause imbalance and disease, and interfere with our ability to fully tap into our power as Creators.

Once I became open to caring for myself, I realized that my lack of energy had several different causes. First, I was constantly focused on getting things done. In fact, I was so busy "doing" all day that I was heading toward full-blown burnout. However, the reason I kept myself so busy wasn't my extensive to-do list; rather, my to-do list was a coping mechanism that protected me from having to feel and deal with any blocked emotions from my earlier life.

For a long time, I was oblivious to these coping mechanisms that kept my emotions undigested. My energy field became heavier and heavier. This culminated in postpartum depression and a deep fear that nothing would ever get better in my life. My circumstances forced me to become more aware of my discomfort, and as a result, I began to "feel."

The dominant emotion was sadness—and much of that sadness was related to my parents' divorce. By denying those feelings for so many years, they had become stuck within me and reinforced a strong sense of feeling unsafe. I was unable to live my life and create a new story because I was stuck in the past.

I was very sad about my parents' divorce. To cope with this uncomfortable feeling, I constructed a story with a happy ending. I told myself that this was the best thing for everyone—that things were fine, and that it would all work out. The problem was, this didn't hold true—at least, not at first. My mother developed a problem with alcohol after the divorce and struggled for many years just to survive. My father was as supportive as he could be in the situation, but he was creating a new life for himself, too. Over time, they both found new partners who seemed to fulfill them, and they both became more balanced. However, undigested pain remained—for them, and for me.

My parents' decision to change their stories changed mine, too. My story of unity and family togetherness was suddenly shattered and replaced by feelings of isolation, insecurity, and fragmentation that were never named or addressed. As the eldest child, I felt responsible for the happiness and well-being of everyone in my family, including my parents, and me and my siblings tried for years to help my mother. At one moment we all realized my mother was not able to continue like this. I must thank my youngest sisters Robin and Deborah for having the courage to instigate an intervention on her behalf. Although my mother didn't live into old age, because of my sisters and the family uniting, she was able at this point to quit drinking forever. For the last years of her life, we enjoyed being with my mother again as she had returned to being her authentic self.

Although my mother healed in many ways, I myself had many unhealed emotions and wounds from all these experiences. After my son's birth, I was so out of balance with these undigested emotions and the physical burnout that I needed to take antidepressants. My psychiatrist explained that my panic attacks were a symptom of postpartum depression and that my brain was working in slow motion. The slow working of my brain made me unable to process scary thoughts and fears, and unfortunately, they began to take over my daily experience. The antidepressants lifted me out of the dark places I was inhabiting, but they were like a Band-Aid placed over a festering wound. On the surface, I was feeling better, but the pills were not helping me to learn how to cope with my difficult stories, undigested emotions, or unhealthy habits and coping mechanisms.

During this time, I met Dr. Nancy Lonsdorf, MD. Trained at Johns Hopkins School of Medicine, she went on to study Ayurvedic medicine, a holistic health and well-being practice developed more than 5,000 years ago by sages in the Indus Valley, and became an integrative physician and bestselling author. She saw that I was "Vata disturbed"—meaning, essentially, that my mind was running wild—and taught me how to meditate, which made a huge difference for me. I also began to eat a nutritious diet and get more exercise. I didn't know it at the time, but meeting Dr. Lonsdorf and incorporating the wellness practices she recommended put me on a path to truly awakening to myself as a spiritual being and a Creator—in part because, by learning to meditate, I learned to confront, digest, and assimilate my stories.

We Are Not Our Stories

Isn't it amazing how we all narrate our own stories? We can tell a story in so many ways, depending on our mood, our self-esteem at any given time, and our perception of how well our life is going at that moment. How we view our stories will impact our self-talk, thoughts, emotions, and choices that continue to steer our destiny.

When our stories are going well, we want to "become" them. We can get lost in the illusion that somehow we are better because our story is turning out so well. However, as our stories make unexpected twists and turns that may not fit as well with our ego and desires, we may wish to distance ourselves from them as much as possible. We can also get lost in the stories that are less flattering and not going so well, which can make us feel stuck and keep us living in the past.

What I have experienced throughout my life is that I am not my story. I am merely *having* a story and co-creating an experience for the sake of my soul's learning and development. The better I become at separating myself from my stories and recognizing that I have a choice in how I feel about them, the freer and less attached to the outcomes I am.

I tell my students the same thing. Over and over, I say, "You are *not* your story." This can be difficult to grasp because our identities get wrapped up in our stories to the point where we can't tell one from the other. Yet, learning to distinguish between who we are and who we tell ourselves we are is one of the most important steps to accessing the Creator Matrix. Creating from our stories will only create more variations of those stories. If we want more or different things for ourselves, we need to detach from the stories so we can create from a different perspective.

Moreover, our stories can lead us to personal judgments and labels that we identify with and hold on to. Examples of this can be the many "I am" statements that we repeat about ourselves, like "I am an addict," "I am a divorcee," "I am sick," "I am forgetful," etc. In my work with clients, my first step has always been to support them to detach from these self-perpetuating statements and then reprogram them. I have noticed that this can be particularly powerful when working with people who have manifested a disease. Once diagnosed, they often use statements like, "I am a cancer patient," "I am diabetic," or "I am a heart patient" when referring to themselves. Helping them return to the core of who they really are helps them break this cycle of attachment. Practicing new "I am" sentences can be very helpful; for example, "I am that I am," or simply, "I am."

What can complicate the process of detachment is that our stories involve others. Our life stories intermingle constantly with the stories of our families, friends, colleagues, and communities. We can become stuck and addicted to the drama of these relationships, and even the dramas of other people. When we recognize that we are not our stories, we can learn to create healthy boundaries and take responsibility for what is ours and what is not.

Learning boundaries should begin in childhood. As I raised my three children, I realized that healthy boundaries kept them safe and empowered them to identify the impact they had on their own environment. Throughout all my years of helping people, I have realized that "being safe" is the critical foundation that most of us must heal. Living in this earthly reality has left many wounds, and as a result, many people feel both unsafe and unsure of how to place boundaries to protect themselves. In order to evolve and understand ourselves as Creators, it is important to also understand how to create safety for ourselves in all situations.

Digesting Our Stories and Experiences

Over my many years of helping people heal, I have realized that the human body is miraculous on all levels of existence. Each part of our bodies serves a purpose. Nothing is in our body by accident. We are very aware of the importance of our senses, like our eyes, ears, taste, smell, and ability to feel. However, realizing that each system plays a role in our ability to manage and maneuver our way through life was like an "a-ha" moment. The digestive system itself is quite extraordinary. Science is showing that our true health begins with this system.

What I have come to understand is that every system exists multidimensionally. The digestive system is also our emotional processing system. Emotions are always our compass, letting us know how we are doing as we are creating and interacting with life.

When difficulties happen in life and we don't understand how to create safety for ourselves, we often search for comfort. Our habits often grow out of our stories, emerging as a way for us to create a sense of safety by distancing ourselves from pain. This process may not always be conscious, as the experience may be too painful, or we might not have the space and time to digest it properly. In this way, habits can also distance us from our emotions while simultaneously feeding our stories.

It has been said, "All good habits have their story." Our habits, while they may seem to support us on the surface, can shield us from the pain of our stories and therefore interfere with our digestion of them.

When we are ready to become co-Creators with Universal Source, we need to observe both our stories and our habits and notice how our habits are serving us in the context of our current stories. Effective observation is the first step in *digesting* what has happened to us; truly taking it in, understanding its meaning, accepting it, assimilating it, and incorporating it into our new consciousness. Without undertaking this process, real change is often not possible—or, at least, it is not sustainable.

You'll notice my emphasis on the term "digestion." Digestion is not only related to digesting actual food but to the processing and integration of all the thoughts, emotions, beliefs, and habits that come out of our life experiences. Just as our digestive system helps us take what we need from our food so our body can function optimally, "digesting" our stories and emotions helps us take what we need from our life experiences, integrate the necessary and desired aspects into our core being, and let go of what is not needed. In this way our digestive system helps us emotionally process. As we learned in Chapter One, all the levels of our being are linked, and work together within our Creator Matrix.

Some people say, "You are what you eat." It would actually be more accurate to say, "You become what you can digest."

When we compartmentalize our experiences from our emotions and develop habits to avoid or minimize them, we are not integrating them. This, as you have seen, creates challenges that can become obstacles to our wellness.

So, how do we begin to "digest" our stories so that we can create a new reality on all levels of being? First, we understand and begin to observe the stages of healthy digestion.

There are four stages of healthy digestion: conscious allowance, acceptance, assimilation, and release.

Conscious Allowance

We begin the process by becoming consciously aware of what we have *allowed* in our life. To be a true Creator, we must become aware that everything and everyone in our matrix is there on some level because we have allowed it to be. As we become conscious of our Creatorship, we take more responsibility for what we have allowed. For example, no one "suddenly" ends up in an unhappy marriage. Such a situation does not just happen to us. On some level, we have allowed it and participated in its co-creation. Only once we make the decision that the marriage is no longer serving us in its current form, and that we will not allow it to continue like this anymore, can we co-create it differently. In a similar way, we have allowed everything and everyone that is participating in our creative story—including challenges to our physical health and well-being. Some of these challenges may not have even originated in this lifetime.

However, everything that is happening to us is showing up as part of our story and, therefore, needs to be resolved and healed on some level.

Sometimes we cannot understand why bad things that create suffering happen. Indeed, many people believe that life simply "happens to" us, without us having any say in the matter. In my experience, the most difficult and darkest times of my life have been the times that helped my soul to grow. While I couldn't see this while in the middle of the story, these experiences were defining moments that shaped who I have become. Perhaps if I had never experienced certain challenges and stories in my youth, I would not be able to help people the way I do now. I encourage you to look at your own stories in the same way. Who have you become as a result of your challenges?

Acceptance

Stage two of healthy digestion is *acceptance*—of both our stories and habits themselves, and of the things we have allowed to unfold within those stories and habits. How easy is it for us to accept all parts of our stories? Some parts of our lives may be easier for us to accept than others. It can be more comfortable to remain in shame, blame, or denial than to fully come to terms with what we have allowed.

This takes practice, and it isn't easy. As we become aware of and accept our own roles in our stories, it's natural to feel the emotions that have gone undigested so far. Lower-frequency emotions like sadness, anger, and frustration may surface. Sometimes, when we realize that we are responsible for allowing a story to occur, or to continue for longer than we wished, we can have feelings of disappointment in ourselves as well.

Here's an example. A man starts a new job and finds himself living in survival mode for many years as the relationship with his boss becomes continually more contentious. There seems to be no time during these years to process and digest the many stressful experiences that have occurred with this boss. The man stays in the job far longer than he wants to because he believes he can't financially afford to quit.

He finally experiences a physical burnout and is forced to leave. As he is recuperating, he feels sadness and disappointment when he thinks about what happened to him. Before he can move on, however, he must focus on the health of his body, mind, and emotional spirit. He finds a therapist who helps him to process and digest his experiences. In particular, she helps him to see what he allowed by staying in that job for too long, and helps him accept the part he played in the relationship with his boss. As he moves into acceptance, he feels anger, sadness, rage, and fear—first at his boss for "doing this" to him, and then at himself for allowing it. Only once these emotions have been felt and digested can he identify what he learned from that experience and choose what he would like to do differently in his next job. To help with this process of digestion, he also joins a gym and begins to meditate. After several months, he is ready to let go, forgive, and move on.

The acceptance stage requires us to not only take responsibility for what we have created but to release ourselves from our stories around that creation. If you're not sure what you are or aren't accepting, just look at your story. Does it leave you feeling powerful or powerless? Are you blaming others for situations you participated in? Are you able to see your own choice points in the narrative? If you are still feeling like your story "happened to" you, are assigning blame, or feeling like you had no choice, those are places to focus your lens of observation.

Several years ago, I received news that my mother was suddenly incoherent and had many brain tumors. I had trouble accepting this new turn of events. This change in my mother's circumstance affected me on all levels of body, mind, and spirit. I didn't want to believe that I would never be able to speak with her normally again. I was suddenly unable to eat and felt nauseous for weeks. Looking back, this was not surprising; when we receive an emotional or mental shock, we often feel it in our stomachs, and it can affect our ability to eat and digest physically.

Unfortunately, my mother passed away not long after that. After returning from the funeral, I developed a terrible stomach virus that caused me to vomit violently for twenty-four hours. What was happening here?

Life events can reverberate throughout our Creator Matrix, impacting all of our systems at all levels of mind, body, and spirit. Because we exist in all dimensions, our experiences affect us multidimensionally. Therefore, our experiences must also be accepted emotionally and spiritually. My sickness was my body's way of "purging" the emotions I did not want to accept. A year later, I worked on healing these emotions with the help of an acupuncturist. This is when I realized that not allowing myself to grieve properly had consequences.

I often ask my clients, "What would it feel like for you if you could accept this?" or "Imagine you could accept this. What would you do then?" However, it's important to note that acceptance is not complacency. We must accept the stories and experiences that we have allowed, but also accept that they are not *us,* and do not change who we are as living expressions of Universal Source. When you reach this place, the emotional and physical charge around the story or habit will dissipate, leaving you feeling relieved, lighter, and free.

Assimilation

Once we have accepted what we have allowed (or are still allowing), we are ready to continue the digestive process through *assimilation.*

Just as our body must choose what it needs from our food in the form of nutrients, vitamins, minerals, and so on, so must we choose what we will learn and can utilize from our life stories as we integrate the beliefs, thoughts, and emotions around them into our being. To some degree, this process actually happens simultaneously to physical digestion; as we digest the foods of the day, we also digest our experiences and the emotions that are showing up alongside our stories. As our food and experiences move through our digestive system, both the nutrients and the lessons learned can be utilized, assimilated, and integrated into our being. And, just as macronutrients and micronutrients are utilized to nurture our cells, which then become our organs, which then become our physical bodies, our digested stories will determine how we express ourselves in the world and our soul evolves.

As we move through the digestive process, we can ask ourselves, taking a helicopter view: "What can I learn from this story, and how can I use what I have learned?"

Release

The final stage of digestion is to release what we do not need.

When we feel unsafe to be who we truly are on Earth, we have trouble letting go because we have not allowed, accepted, and assimilated all aspects of ourselves. When we aren't free to be who we are, we often distrust our inner voice and therefore fail to listen to the intuitive messages that our body gives us.

On a physical level, we release what we don't need via our bladder, colon, sweat, and mucus. We often don't take the time to nurture this process by drinking enough water, exercising, breathing properly, and simply taking the time to sit on the toilet to release. Becoming conscious of giving ourselves space and time to release what we don't need on all levels is very important. When the body feels unsafe—either because of our stories or because of a current situation—it will have trouble letting go of what it doesn't need. Over the years, we may have held onto particular emotions, thereby slowing our digestion. The consequence is that food becomes older, more toxic, and the intestines can become inflamed. Many people who are uncomfortable being their true selves can experience chronic constipation.

I often encourage my students to get into the habit of talking to their bodies daily. One way to begin is to repeat the following statement: "I give my body permission to release all that does not serve me anymore." As we learn to observe our own stories and subconscious, we can work with our bodies to truly let go of all we no longer require to thrive.

Feeding Our Stories: Primary and Secondary Food

Among my other certifications, I'm a graduate of the Institute for Integrative Nutrition (IIN). Their base philosophy is the importance of "primary food"—meaning, how a person nourishes and sustains themselves in all areas of life, including career, home life, relationships, social life, education, spirituality, finances, sleep, rest, and life goals. These areas of life lay the foundation for and influence our relationship with food itself. The *actual* food we eat is termed "secondary food."

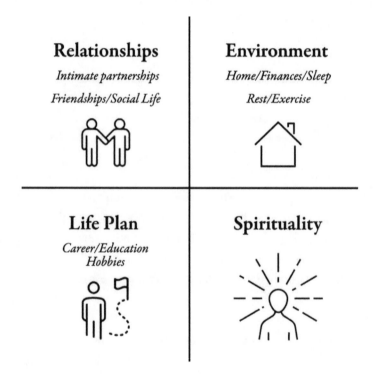

Relationships
Intimate partnerships
Friendships/Social Life

Environment
Home/Finances/Sleep
Rest/Exercise

Life Plan
Career/Education
Hobbies

Spirituality

All areas of our lives influence and interact with each other. We are often unaware of the connection between our life stories and the food we eat. As mentioned above, digestion can happen by physically eating food, which helps us process our stories both emotionally and mentally as well. When we look at the body, mind, and spirit matrix holistically, we see that learning to care for all areas of our life is fundamental for our health and well-being.

As we learn to become our Creator-selves, we can consciously choose which areas of life to nurture. This is fundamental to claiming ownership of our creative process. When we are living in survival mode, we don't realize which areas of life are potentially impacting our Creator Matrix. We are living life unaware and disconnected. As we become more conscious, we realize that we are responsible for all areas of our lives. We can then choose which areas need more attention and which already feel well-nourished, and adapt our habits and patterns accordingly. This will consequently help us to create a more robust and individualized definition of self-care. The science of epigenetics, which we will explore in Chapter Seven, is proving the power of our choices.

Conscious manifesting involves active participation. Therefore, it is important to explore which areas feel out of balance and in need of change. Once these areas enter our awareness, we can take action to implement the changes we desire. These action steps may focus on changing a storyline in any primary or secondary food area. Perhaps some habits may also need to be reevaluated and restructured. Understanding this as the Creator of our lives means choosing what will be nourished and when, as nourishment is essential to all areas of life itself.

Up until now, many of us have been trying to nourish ourselves through outside influences—like people, food, the accumulation of material possessions, travel, money, and social media likes, to name but a few. As we grow and become more holistically minded, we realize that, as multidimensional beings, we need to nourish all aspects of ourselves. The core of self-nourishment is our body, mind, and spirit matrix—our Creator Matrix. Once this matrix functions optimally, we will come into full power as Creators.

This is all about becoming more committed to our own wellness, happiness, and self-fulfillment. During the process, we may become aware of the fear and judgments we have about ourselves and life in general. Everything we fear and judge will show up repeatedly until acceptance can take place. Acceptance is what brings our energetic system into balance and back to a "neutral point." It is more difficult to create what we want from a space of "standing against," rather than from a place of "standing for." We attract to us what we fear and judge because the energy wants to be healed. Moreover, learning to develop ourselves as non-judgmental observers—including our stories, digestion, and primary and secondary food choices—will quicken the process of change. Ultimately, acceptance is about learning to truly love who we are unconditionally. It is only through this unconditional self-love that we can truly become nourished.

Nourishing the Body, Mind, and Spirit

How we view our body and the feelings we have about it is extremely important in what kind of health we create for ourselves.

We all have a relationship with our bodies. In our DNA, we have cellular memories and genetic influences of experiences that might not have been so safe for our bodies. These experiences may have been ours, or they may have belonged to our ancestors and been passed down to us. Pain brings discomfort, concern, and stress that can influence these cellular memories. These memories, conscious or subconscious, might keep us from fully embracing our bodies and loving them.

What would real love for our bodies look like? I think it would start with trusting them. The trust frequency is one of the highest frequencies that exists. The vibration of trust brings us in alignment with ourselves. When we trust our bodies, we can hear and listen to what they need.

Our bodies also pick up information from our environment and relationships. Are we safe or not safe? Relaxed or tense? If we are under stress or duress, our muscles tighten and vital functions slow or shut down. If we are uncomfortable or surrounded by mess or chaos, we will not rest well. If we are not spiritually connected to nature and Universal Source (in whatever ways feel aligned to us), our bodies may feel heavy and detached from the world around us. If we are not moving our bodies, our emotional and mental processing and digestion likewise slows down.

And then, of course, there's food.

Food—which, remember, is "secondary food" for our Creator Matrix—is energy and has information for our bodies. It *becomes* us. When we eat, we bring nourishment in from outside ourselves; not only does it give us energy, but it also builds and repairs every single cell in our bodies. Remember, we become what we eat and can digest.

Caring for our cellular health is an important aspect of physical nourishment. What do I mean by cellular health? Everything! One important aspect is how we provide (secondary food) nutrition to our bodies to have the building blocks available for replacing around 330 billion cells per day—or 1 percent of our body. Our bodies need the right components to build proper structure, which affects function. How well your body can continually rejuvenate will determine how you age, how and when you get sick, and your overall physical resilience.

Eating the right macro- and micronutrients is essential for optimal cell communication and function. To maintain a healthy system on all levels of body, mind, and spirit, cells must be able to clean themselves (detox), as well as build and repair every day. Healthy cells do what we do when we are healthy: they allow, accept, assimilate, and then release what they no longer need (toxins) into the tissue, lymph, and circulatory systems. This process keeps your whole system connected and in constant communication. When the physical body becomes too toxic at the cellular level, the energetic body is affected. Similarly, when the energetic body is blocked by undigested emotions, the cells and tissues can also be impacted. In this way, the system can become blocked both physically and energetically, drastically reducing our ability to harness the power and connectivity of our Creator Matrix.

For our bodies to be well, our minds and emotions must also be in balance. The aspects of body, mind, and spirit are connected and influence each other at the cellular level. How balanced and happy we are in the realm of our primary foods will often influence the secondary food choices we make. You likely know that there is a connection between being emotionally unhappy and unhealthy eating. (It's called "comfort food" for a reason!) Sometimes, this connection between emotions and eating serves a purpose; it is a way of comforting ourselves when we aren't sure how to digest the ways in which life is impacting us. When we own our Creatorship, we acknowledge that, on some level, we have allowed and chosen our primary and secondary foods. How we love ourselves, and how conscious we become of this relationship between primary and secondary foods, will impact the kinds of choices we make. I see in my coaching practice how, once people start making changes in one area, it often creates a ripple effect, and changes occur in other areas. Therefore, nourishing our minds and spirits is a vital counterpart to nourishing our bodies. Learning how to love and care for all aspects of our bodies will provide an important foundation for both creating multidimensional wellness and expanding our consciousness.

How do we nourish our mind and spirit? With thoughts and emotions. For this reason, it is important to look at which thoughts, feelings, and emotions we are giving priority to. What we focus on will expand. Where we put our energy will determine where, and how, we are nourished. When we become aware of what we think about all day long, we begin to realize how our thoughts influence our lives. The mind is often a chaotic place, and many of us are suffering from information overload. This overload may be intensified by the negative news we watch and listen to, the devices we are attached to, or just the daily demands and stresses of life. However, most of us are not aware of how chaotic our mental state is becoming.

Thoughts are real, and we can refer to them as "thought forms." They exist despite us not being able to see them with our eyes. They induce biochemical and electrical conduction through the neurons to all the cells of the body. Just like a computer, the more input coming into the system, the more vulnerable we are to overload or burnout. On the other hand, the more balanced our brains, the better we can create, manage, and process our thoughts. We will begin to explore how our thoughts and feelings influence our bodies at an energetic and cellular level in Chapter Six.

Balancing Yang and Yin Energies to Manifest within Your Creator Matrix

As a Creator, we become conscious of using two different energetic forces. These energetic forces, otherwise known as "yang" and "yin," correspond with the cycles of manifesting and digestion.

Yang and yin energies, like masculine and feminine energies, exist in all of us and correspond to natural cycles. We have both, and we need both. However, most of us tend to favor one over the other.

Yang energy, which is sometimes associated with the masculine, is an "active" energy. It is the process of manifestation. It begins with a thought or intention. Perhaps you identify something that you want to do or create. You make a goal, consciously or unconsciously, to carry out this idea (for example, applying to a school, seeking out a new job, joining a dating site, writing a book, etc.). You make a plan and begin to act, step by step, to create the desire you have identified. With this outward focus, you begin to see something manifest; each step leads toward the next. Eventually, as you stick it out, your dream becomes a reality.

Yang energy is highly prized in our world. It's "doer" energy. However, what is often not understood is that this is not where the story of creation ends.

In order to fully experience and learn from what you have created, it's important to enter the other phase, Yin, which allows the space to digest, integrate, learn, and become. This is where our process of digestion occurs. If Yang energy is hunting, skinning, roasting, and eating the food, yin is sitting around the fire after the meal, digesting and telling stories. Yin energy also involves feelings, which help us to mirror our experiences from all angles, understand what roles we have played and how we have reacted to challenges along the way, and ultimately integrate what we have experienced to become a new version of ourselves.

Together, yang and yin form a complete cycle of creation. As we move through one creation cycle after another, our consciousness is constantly evolving.

The Yang/Yin Cycle

YANG — MANIFESTING	YIN — DIGESTION
Characteristics: • Pushes outward • Light/bright • Doing/acting • Giving	**Characteristics:** • Pulls inward • Dark • Feeling/sensing • Receiving
Examples: • Speaking • Exercising • Taking action/ expressing	**Examples:** • Sleeping • Meditating • Reflecting/ observing

Balancing our own yang and yin energies is a highly individual process. For some, this means engaging in regular vigorous exercise, spending time in public places, or knocking items off a to-do list. For others, it could mean meditation, yoga, breathwork, or taking a long walk in nature. The objective is not to "cancel out" your dominant energy, but to give your mind, body, and spirit the support they need to move through creation cycles with greater ease, fluidity, and attention. When this happens, well-being is achieved.

Personally, I have always felt more comfortable in the active Yang energy of life. However, as I shared at the beginning of this chapter, I experienced a burnout period after the birth of my son. I felt overwhelmed, exhausted, and sad. I didn't realize that my brain and my neurotransmitters had reached a crisis point. Once I understood what was happening, I changed not only the ways in which I was caring for my body, mind, and spirit in the short term, but also my longer-term work-life balance. The result was that I had a very different experience throughout the pregnancies, births, and postpartum periods with my two younger children. I worked much less during the pregnancies, watched what I ate, took prenatal yoga classes, and meditated every day. After both births, I participated in an Ayurvedic Mom and Baby program, received regular massages for just a few weeks, and used various other self-care practices. The result was that I not only felt good but also truly enjoyed the postpartum period with my daughters. My mind felt calm and clear, and my emotions were mostly happy. Spiritually, I felt very grateful and connected to motherhood. My daughters received the benefits of my balanced state. Unlike my son's challenging and turbulent beginning, my daughters were healthy, balanced, and thriving.

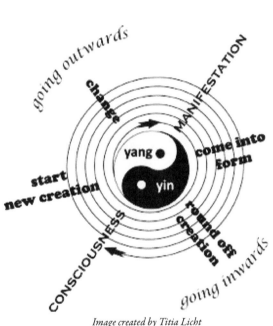

Image created by Titia Licht

The Science of The Creator Process

We will be exploring the science behind manifesting in the chapters to come, but it's important to know that the basic premise of quantum physics is that we are all connected to a quantum field or Universal

Field, and that we can influence this field and change our materialistic world. Nassim Haramein, a researcher, physicist, and speaker, believes that consciousness has an impact on matter. According to Haramein, "Consciousness, matter, space, and gravity influence each other within a unified, interactive field."[1]

As a Creator, we realize that our thoughts influence the field and our manifestations. Becoming aware of the Law of Allowing can help us to take ownership of what we have manifested and would like to manifest. Many of my students over the years have created great change in their lives by simply observing what they have allowed in their life. By accepting this responsibility, they take another great step toward owning their creative power. Once you realize that you have allowed everything in your life, the house, the relationships, the job, the drama, the choices, and how you react to what happens, the more you own your own power rather than be a victim of it. Science is showing us that through our thoughts and intentions we consciously or unconsciously affect the Universal Field. The more conscious we become of our thoughts and intentions, and the more aligned they become with the body, mind, and spirit complex, the quicker those thoughts and intentions will manifest.

Once you think a thought and it transmits to the etheric field, this thought is instantly manifested in the etheric plane. In the old, dense energy of the past, we often got sidetracked at this point by life itself and we stopped focusing on our initial desire or intention as it seemed almost impossible to manifest anymore. There have always been a few people in the old energy who remained focused and had enough faith in themselves and in the process to manifest despite the obstacles. With the new energy bandwidth on the planet at this time, the Creator Process (as shown in the diagram below) is much easier. Many might understand this described process, but their Creator Matrix is not yet in alignment with their heart's desires. What they have intended to create is not showing up because they are misaligned. They will need to focus on removing what is not serving them on all levels of body, mind, and spirit to create a match of frequency in their Creator Matrix. Once your matrix is aligned, manifesting will be like connecting one's radio station to the perfect channel. Communication will be coherent and divine synchronicities will start to show up. Then it becomes your responsibility to consciously focus on the opportunities the universe will be sending your way.

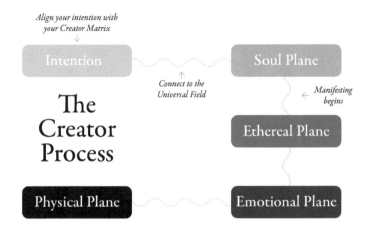

Manifesting is like a co-creative dance between you, Prime Creator, and the field of creation (Universal Source). Once you focus, you will begin to see the opportunities that are being presented. For some, it will feel like a coincidence at first; however, after a while, you will note these as synchronicities of your creation. It will then become important to take rightful action to take the steps to make the opportunity happen. I built my business in this way. I had no idea how to do it. I just started and I was completely guided along these lines. For example, one day I noticed that in my email box was an invitation to join the National Board of Health and Wellness Coaching. I thought at that moment I would like my students to have this opportunity. Then over the next months the organization kept showing up in different places. Until one day I noticed in my email a message from the National Board, last chance to apply. Covid happened two weeks later and gave me the opportunity to complete the application for my organization. These kinds of stories kept repeating day after day, month after month, year after year, and I kept showing up focused and ready—until now, years later, I have built a wonderful coaching institute, and my dream has been manifested.

We are indeed awakening to our true power as human beings: that we are Creators. As we connect to this consciousness of why we are here on Earth and who we are, we will begin to learn how to manifest effortlessly and easily. This process takes practice, and we need patience with ourselves. I have learned that we can become more powerful Creators learning to manifest and digest when we make it a priority to consciously create health and wellness on all levels of our Creator Matrix. It can be challenging to be a Creator when we don't feel well. Over time, we will learn to perfect our abilities to co-create with ourselves on both energetic and cellular levels, with each other, and with all that is through the Universal Field. As Creators, we will learn to use our creativity in this process. Each of us will connect with our divine Creator within and learn to see and appreciate the Creator in all those we co-create with. We will start to see the beauty in the uniqueness of each soul.

Next, we will look at how each person has been given their own unique template as a base from which to create.

Chapter Summary

- Our stories are the first point of attention when we begin to work within our Creator Matrix and explore full-spectrum wellness.

- Our stories touch, influence, and shape everything about our multidimensional selves.

- We need to learn to identify, digest, and consciously shape our stories, which starts with self-reflection.

- During our first seven years, we develop many of the beliefs, values, and habits that guide us throughout our lives.

- We are Creators and we make things happen in our lives through our actions, reactions, responses, and beliefs, driven by our stories.

- We are not our stories. We are *having* our stories and co-creating an experience for our soul's learning and development.

- We need to detach from our stories so we can create from a different perspective. The better we become at separating ourselves from our stories and recognizing that we have a choice in how we feel about them, the freer and less attached to the outcomes we are.

- When we recognize that we are not our stories, we can learn to create healthy boundaries and take responsibility for what is ours and what is not.

- Our habits often grow out of our stories, emerging as a way for us to create a sense of safety by distancing ourselves from pain.

- We need to digest the stories, experiences, emotions, and habits we've been living with subconsciously until now.

- There are four stages of healthy digestion: conscious allowance, acceptance, assimilation, and release.

- Once we have digested everything until now, we can begin to make more conscious decisions about what we will digest and how we feed and nourish our body, mind, and spirit.

- We are learning to take responsibility for what we have allowed in our lives (Law of Allowing), the house, the relationships, the job, the drama, the choices, and how we react to what happens.

- We can nourish our bodies by loving and trusting our bodies, by caring for our cellular health via the food we eat and keeping our minds and emotions in balance.

- Two energies exist in all of us, yin and yang, corresponding with the cycles of manifesting and digestion, together forming a complete cycle of creation.

- It is a highly individual process to balance yin and yang energy in order to move through creation cycles with greater ease, fluidity, and attention, achieving more well-being.

- As a Creator we can consciously influence the Universal Field and manifest via our thoughts and intentions. We will do this unconsciously until we make this process conscious. We will learn to align our creative intentions with the unified field and bring into physical form that which we wish to manifest.

Chapter Three

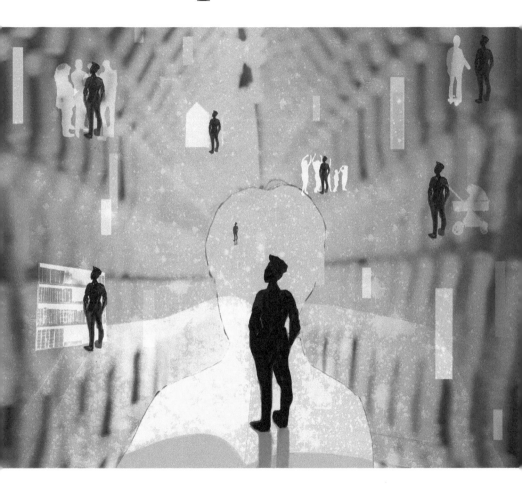

How well do you know yourself and how unique you are?

"Knowing yourself is the beginning of all wisdom."

- Aristotle

CHAPTER THREE

Our Unique Templates and Storylines

W e are all unique. Our uniqueness creates the magic between us and influences our creativity and co-creations.

As a nurse, I helped many people cope with the reality of their illnesses or ailments. Working with patients, I learned that each soul has different perspectives and many different influences upon them that tremendously impact how they will navigate a given situation. The beauty and uniqueness of each human soul is a gift. What binds us together is that we are all Creators.

As we observe the different choices of others and become part of their stories, we see that although each soul has been given the same basic template to create from, they inevitably choose different paths that are influenced by their authentic natures. As we grow in consciousness, we will choose different paths that influence how the unique template of "us" will expand and evolve. Imagine if we really were all exactly the same. How boring and limited our creations would be!

In my large Catholic family, we were raised with many beliefs about many things. We were told that to "believe" was right and good. Moreover, we were taught to believe in a power higher than ourselves, with which we as human beings are interconnected. To have this belief system gave us confidence that this "higher power" was somehow guiding and looking out for us. This belief had many advantages for me, as my faith always empowered me to pull myself out of desperate situations. However, the illusion was that this "higher power" was outside of myself. This often left me with feelings of judgment, guilt, and shame when I felt I had made a mistake in my life choices and decisions. My family in particular was also taught that we needed to help the disadvantaged people around us. If we did not do this, we couldn't consider ourselves to be "good" or righteous. I have since learned that this is common for many who are raised in religious households.

It wasn't until I was in my thirties, after having moved to the Netherlands, that I started to realize that a belief was not a fact. Furthermore, not only was a belief not a fact, but it might not even be a belief that originated with me! I started to ask questions and explore what this "higher power" really meant to me and how it would serve my life. I began to study various religions and found a common thread of faith, belief, and service in all of them. I realized that my relationship with this "higher power" was an internal process that was non-judgmental and very loving.

Over time, it became increasingly clear to me that many of the beliefs I had held for my whole life were no longer serving me. Many "truths" that I had assumed were unassailable also no longer felt aligned.

One particular example comes to mind. I was raised with the belief that it was not good to pursue making money for the sake of making money. It was far better to pursue a career in the field of education, service, and intellectual development, as those careers were seen as being in service to others. People who "just made money" were seen as somehow less worthy, and even as selfish or unethical. Having been raised with this belief, I always felt guilty about having money, and for wanting to create a life where there was enough money. However, as I met more people from different backgrounds and walks of life, I began to see that people who had money and made a lot of money were also wonderful people. I began to question this very limited belief. Then, one day, I thought, "I don't actually believe this." For the first time I could remember, I consciously let go of a belief that was no longer serving me. From that moment onward, I began a new relationship with money and abundance.

As human beings living on Planet Earth, we have beliefs about *everything*. We have beliefs about ourselves, our health and wellness, our values, our worthiness, our abilities, our talents, our strengths and weaknesses, our families, our communities, and about the world as a whole and our place in it. Many beliefs are so strong that they amount to programming; meaning, they underpin, influence, and even control our self-talk and much of our behavior. Therefore, as we are learning to work within our Creator Matrix and consciously design our lives, it makes sense that we should pay attention to what our beliefs are, how they are created, and how we can change them when they are no longer working for us.

Merriam-Webster defines a belief as "something that is accepted, considered to be true, or held as an opinion: something believed especially: a tenet or body of tenets held by a group."[1]

This particular definition of belief reinforced my consciousness of how beliefs influence our motivations, perceptions, and actions. If the belief is only a concept that one holds as true but is not necessarily true, the next question is, "What is truth"?

To answer that question—"What is truth?"—was much more difficult for me. Over time, I have realized that everyone has their own beliefs, and those beliefs form their own truths. Those truths, perhaps, may not be absolute, but that doesn't make them less "true" to those who hold them.

If we believe something, does that make it true? Well, we may think so—but, objectively, that is not necessarily the case. If two people have opposing beliefs, then they can't *both* be true, no matter how fervently each person holds their individual beliefs. However, they *can* be true for the individuals, even if they are untrue for others.

This realization has helped me develop a compassion for humanity. It also prompted me to create a process that I still use today: a habit of critically observing my beliefs.

To do this, I ask myself three questions:

1. Is this belief true to me?

2. Is this belief "from" me? Is it really mine?

3. Does this belief still serve me?

All of us pick up beliefs in life through our experiences, things we are told, and conclusions we reach in relation to our life stories. Our beliefs, therefore, are subjective and also reflective of our relationship to our environment and the people around us. They are not part of our "nature," but of our "nurturing." And, until we recognize that they are not absolute, our beliefs can dominate our lives without us even knowing it.

There are people who believe the world is a scary place filled with "bad" people. There are others who believe that the world is a wonderful place filled with good people. Who is correct? Actually, in a way, they both are. Once a belief becomes embedded in our subconscious, it acts as a programming tool for producing behavior patterns that are consistent with that belief. So, people who hold the former belief will operate from a place of fear, always on the defensive, and make decisions in their lives and relationships that reflect that "scary" world. People who hold the latter belief will operate from a place of love and curiosity, which will also be reflected in their experiences and relationships. Of course, regardless of our beliefs, there are real dangers in our world that call for caution. However, fear has a tendency to become exacerbated and irrational, especially when it becomes entangled with beliefs. For example, when someone who thinks the world is a scary place watches the mainstream news every day, they will receive confirmation that they should be afraid, even if the news has no direct bearing on their lives. In that way, our beliefs become self-fulfilling prophecies, and end up reinforcing themselves through our stories and perceptions.

As we are awakening, we start to recognize our limiting beliefs. What are limiting beliefs? They are thoughts about ourselves and the world around us that can restrict us and our lives. They can keep us from owning our true power as a Creator. They come from fears and protection and can also be passed on through the DNA and ancestral lineages and reside in the subconscious.

Some common limiting beliefs that may need to be released at this time include:

- I am not good enough.

- I do not matter.

- There is not enough time.

- I will never have enough money.

- I will never be happy.

Many of our limiting beliefs will need to be reprogrammed. My initial experience with reprogramming some of my own limiting beliefs was with José the kinesiologist. Later I began to work with a technique known as EFT (Emotional Freedom Technique). These techniques help the body, mind, and spirit matrix of each Creator become aligned with the highest expression of their creations.

Becoming more conscious of our limiting beliefs will help us clear out the cobwebs in the subconscious. However, in addition to subconscious influences, many people also consciously focus on what they don't want every day. It is therefore important to become aware of what you are focusing on consciously. One helpful exercise can be to write out a list of everything in your life that you don't want but that is currently showing up. Then, take each of those items and write out what you *do* want. For example, if you are constantly sick and focused on your ill health all the time (thereby continually manifesting more ill health), you can begin to change the patterning in your consciousness by imagining yourself healthy and feeling great every day.

In life, it is probable that we will encounter situations that challenge our beliefs. If we fail to consciously become aware of our limiting beliefs, we will feel discomfort or resistance. "Cognitive dissonance" is the term that refers to the mental discomfort that arises from simultaneously holding two contradictory beliefs (for example, when you believe that it's important to teach your children healthy life habits and simultaneously believe that it's acceptable to smoke a cigarette in front of them). When the discomfort of cognitive dissonance becomes great enough, something must change to relieve the nagging feeling. This could be a change in attitude, beliefs, or even values. As a person becomes more conscious, this incongruence of behavior and belief could influence their habits and actions (for example, the choice to finally quit smoking).

As we step into our power as Creators, we need to take responsibility for our own beliefs and see them as bio-individual aspects of our being that are unique and distinctive to us. When we realize that our beliefs don't need to remain static, that we can change them; this gives us the power to change many other aspects of our lives as well, including our emotional states. Our wellness, like our bio-individuality, is an accumulation of life choices that reflect our beliefs. Therefore, when we change our beliefs, we can begin to change our lives.

Beliefs and the Creator Cycle

In Chapter Two, we explored the Yang/Yin Cycle and learned that the process of manifestation is not complete until we have allowed enough time to digest our experiences and learn from them. Both manifestation and digestion must take place in order to complete the cycle. However, when we add beliefs into the mix—particularly beliefs that are fear-based or that contradict what we want to create—our creation cycles can be disrupted and remain unfinished.

Many of us live our lives having new experiences, creating new stories, making new goals ... and never creating any meaningful change. Somehow, somewhere, we have developed patterns that block us from fully digesting our life experiences. These patterns can become habits, but they are rooted in our beliefs.

Self-sabotage is an easy pit to fall into. Better to stay small and safe than to take on more responsibility and get noticed; better to stay safe in your house than interact with people who might harm you; better to start five things at once than put all your energy into one thing that might actually work; better to numb with food or alcohol than to feel those challenging emotions; better to take care of others than take care of ourselves; better to dream than to do. When our feelings from our life stories are intense, they can influence or reinforce our deeply held beliefs about our worth and our deservingness of love.

BELIEFS RESIDE IN THE SUBCONSCIOUS

The Yang/Yin Cycle and the digestion of our emotions and experiences are not the only aspects that influence our creative processes. We are also influenced by our conscious, subconscious, and unconscious states. For the purposes of this discussion, the subconscious and unconscious are interchangeable and infer that, on some level, there is an absence of awareness. Freud talked about the mental mind and the power of these three states of consciousness; he described the mind as being like an iceberg, with only one-seventh of its bulk above the water.[2]

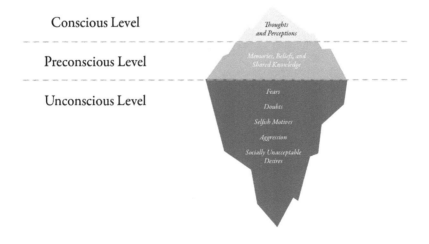

Conscious Level — Thoughts and Perceptions

Preconscious Level — Memories, Beliefs, and Shared Knowledge

Unconscious Level — Fears, Doubts, Selfish Motives, Aggression, Socially Unacceptable Desires

One of my first challenges with regard to becoming the Creator of my life was understanding how powerful my thoughts were in my creations. I realized early on that my thoughts were linked to emotions and feelings, and these feelings seemed to be influenced by my past experiences and directly linked to my future visions, goals, choices, and experiences that I would attract. As I reflected on these visions and past experiences, I became aware of the fears and blocked emotions that were connected to them.

This leads me to my second challenge: recognizing the power of the subconscious.

What is the difference between the conscious and the subconscious? Many people understand the differences between the two on an intellectual level yet are still unable to utilize the information to create their preferred reality. I was completely intent on manifesting the reality I dreamed of, and so I became determined to figure it out. I wanted to understand why the reality that I did *not* dream of kept on showing up. Over time, I began to understand the different facets that were influencing my conscious and subconscious states. In fact, the most powerful force on the creations that were showing up for me seemed to be originating from my subconscious.

Research shows that the conscious mind influences approximately 10 percent of our reality, compared with the subconscious which affects the remaining 90 percent of our creations. The conscious mind can be active in the present, past, and future; it controls our reasoning, perceptions, decisions, conscious thoughts, and recent memories. This conscious state has the greatest effect on our free will. In the conscious state, people can get stuck thinking about their unhappy past, which can lead to depression, or they can get stuck worrying about the future and become overwhelmed with anxiety. However, because the conscious state is, well, conscious, it can seem easier to identify the problem areas, including the beliefs and emotions that underpin the challenging thoughts and behaviors, and work to shift them.

CONSCIOUS (10 PERCENT)	SUBCONSCIOUS (90 PERCENT)	UNCONSCIOUS
Past, present, and future	Programming	Deeper fears
Reasoning	Belief systems	Unacceptable desires and urges
Decision-making	Recordings	Repressed memories and traumas
A person's free will	Past memories (experiences/traumas)	
Conscious thoughts	Present time only (The now!)	
Perceptions	Stored knowledge	
Recent memories	Involuntary actions	
	Fears	

The subconscious state, on the other hand, functions in the present moment only, like a recording that is constantly on autopilot. What gets stored in the subconscious will affect us and our creative process if we are unaware of what "programs" are running in the background.

What kinds of programs hinder our full expression and self-actualization through our Creator Matrix? Limiting beliefs and low-frequency emotions stored in the subconscious are connected to undigested life experiences, fears, and traumas.

The ancient Greeks and Egyptians used forms of self-hypnosis and sought out healers to help people change their unhealthy inner programming. Today, we have many forms of energy medicine and science-based therapies that can help people reprogram the subconscious—including Eye movement desensitization and reprocessing (EMDR), Emotional Freedom Technique (EFT), kinesiology, and Psych-K, to name a few.

Through my work with José and my use of EFT, I have managed to reprogram my subconscious patterns and release many unhelpful beliefs, emotions, and connected life storylines that were impacting my ability to manifest the life I desired. Since addressing these subconscious beliefs, my ability to manifest has become faster and easier. My daily habits, like meditation, chanting, and prayer, have helped me keep my conscious state more in the present moment, objectively observe and evaluate my beliefs, and continue to shift my programming where necessary.

As we become more aware of ourselves as Creators, we start to connect with the wonder and magic of life. We awaken to more connections and possibilities. We can then begin to recreate ourselves and our lives, and literally reinvent our belief systems from the ground up. This, in turn, will influence and change how we narrate our stories, which in turn will change our behaviors and choices. As we learn to observe, shift, and eventually master our beliefs, we will use our thoughts more consciously and be able to move through our emotions more easily. We will recognize our power and use it for the benefit of the whole as we realize that everything is connected.

Our Personality: A Gift and a Lesson

For each of us, the road to well-being and true Creatorship is different. We are not only biologically unique; our thoughts, feelings, emotions, and memories are all distinct.

Each of us has a unique personality that acts as a prism through which we view and experience our lives. Some of us are extroverts, others introverts. Some are filled with athletic prowess, active and energetic, while others are passive, uncoordinated, or reflective. Some are highly intellectual, while others are masterfully creative. Some are fun-loving and full of laughs, whereas others take life so seriously that they never crack a joke. None of these are good or bad, they are simply unique expressions of creation.

In addition to our unique physical forms, stories, and beliefs, we each have our own personality type. It is part of our bio-individuality, and plays a large role in where, when, why, and how we create our reality. As such, it behooves us to know ourselves, accept ourselves for who and what we are, and work with our unique personality rather than fighting against it.

According to the American Psychological Association, personality is defined as "individual differences in characteristic patterns of thinking, feeling, and behaving."[3] However, we often see personalities getting lumped into groups or labeled in various ways based on shared patterns or routines. For example, there is the distinction between Type A (ambitious, meticulous, driven, tend to "live to work") and Type B (relaxed, fun-loving, tend to "work to live") personalities. These distinctions tell us something about ourselves that we probably already know, but also give us a sense of belonging to a group.

People often get labeled as one personality type or another based on their life patterns or routines, even though these may be temporary or context dependent. The key to self-awareness is the willingness to discover our behavioral patterns and how our personality types affect our relationship to ourselves and others, both from moment to moment and in the longer term.

There are different ways to dissect personality as a concept, and it is important to make a distinction between personality and consciousness. As we grow in consciousness, we become more understanding and accepting of how our personality affects ourselves and others. We become more introspective and self-reflective and begin to work on creating more harmony between ourselves and others with different personalities. The greatest realization for many people is recognizing that people are programmed differently based on their unique personality makeup. Although we are often attracted to others who are different from us ("opposites attract"), eventually these differences may become conflictual. Many people in relationships try to change the other to become more like them instead of learning to accept the other as they are without judgment. However, because we are all living and creating according to our own individual beliefs, truths, stories, and personalities, it can be difficult for us to accept differences in each other, and this can create the illusion of "separateness" or disconnection.

What we are learning through evolution and science is that we are all united and connected as aspects of Prime Creator, and our differences are necessary for our growth and expression. When confronted with someone's differences (i.e., different opinions, preferences, choices, values, cultures, language, wavelengths, needs, or levels of consciousness), we therefore have two choices: we can resist these differences, or we can accept them. When we choose to accept them, this may help us transcend them.

HOW DOES THE ENNEAGRAM WORK?

In understanding my own personality and that of others, I have found the Enneagram to be both profound and transformational. This way of looking at personality was brought to the West by George Gurdjieff in 1915. The Enneagram comes from the Greek words *ennea*, meaning nine, and *grammos*, referring to a written or drawn symbol. Russ Hudson, in his foreword to the book *Keys to the Enneagram* by A. H. Almaas, writes: "The Enneagram in its original sense was never meant to be a 'filing system' for human beings ... These type patterns do not reflect our true identity. It would be more accurate to say that awareness of the type pattern can potentially awaken us to the more profound realization of who or what we are beyond all of these patterns."[4]

The Enneagram was created to guide each soul to explore the personality type they chose before being incarnated on Earth. Essentially, it is one influence upon the base template for how they will navigate and interact with the outer and inner world. Each type has different lessons to learn; once the lesson is achieved, they can move beyond their personality constraints.

Our personalities can influence us, but they are not the only influence, nor are they fixed. As we observe ourselves more clearly, old, outdated belief systems can be released; this raises the potential for a more holistic, loving, and accepting view of both the personality and the self as a whole. Learning about their unique personality can guide people toward a deeper reflection of their behavior, motivation, and habits; in particular, the Enneagram can encourage a person's spiritual awakening through self-awareness. In my experience, it has helped me to bring more humor into my interactions with people as I understand the nuanced differences between us all.

According to the Enneagram Theory, there are nine basic personality types. Each of these types has different traits and different life themes. For example, I learned that I was a Type 3 personality (with a Type 2 wing). As a child and young adult, I was anxious and fearful about failing, and I was very concerned about how I came across to others. When I learned that overcoming a fear of failing is the journey of a Type 3, it explained a great deal about my own reactions and behavior to things and situations. This, in turn, helped me to love myself more and, therefore, laugh at myself more.

Each Enneagram type has a positive side and a "shadow" side (core wounds). Moreover, each type tends to use distinct defense mechanisms that help their "shadow" sides cope with life's challenges. It is instructive to look closely at the descriptions that explain this, as they may provide insight into your strengths, your habitual behaviors, and any beliefs that might be influencing your creations, and help you more mindfully navigate your fears, limitations, and areas of self-growth. Underpinning the defense mechanisms are the wounded aspects of each type and what each type needs to overcome and develop toward.

On the next page is a chart of the nine Enneagram personality types, key attributes, and defense mechanisms, adapted from materials created by The Enneagram Institute and Ginger Lapid-Bogda.[5][6]

TYPE	QUALITIES/TRAITS	DEFENSE MECHANISMS/ CORE WOUNDS
1 The Reformer (Rational, idealistic)	Seeks perfection Avoids making mistakes	Reaction formation: tries to reduce/eliminate anxiety *"It's not okay to make mistakes or be wrong."*
2 The Helper (Caring, interpersonal)	Seeks appreciation and feeling needed Avoids feeling unworthy	Repression: hides information about self from self *"It's not okay to have my own needs."*
3 The Achiever (Success oriented, pragmatic)	Seeks respect and admiration Avoids failure	Identification: unconsciously incorporates attributes of another to increase self-esteem *"It's not okay to fail."*
4 The Individualist (Sensitive, withdrawn)	Expresses deep feelings and connections with others Avoids rejection yet wants to be different	Introjection: instead of repelling critical information and negative experiences, fully absorbs them into sense of self *"It's not okay to not fit in."* *"It's not okay to be too emotional."*
5 The Investigator (Intense, cerebral)	Seeks knowledge and wisdom Avoids intrusion by others and loss of energy	Isolation: avoids feeling overwhelmed and empty by isolating themselves and cutting themselves off from their feelings and other people *"I don't have the skills to make it."* *"It's not okay to feel/be (comfortable) in the world."*
6 The Loyalist (Committed, security orientated)	Seeks meaning, certainty, and trust. Avoids negative scenarios from occurring	Projection: attributes their own unacceptable thoughts, emotions, motivations, attributes, and behaviors to others *"It's not okay to trust myself and/or the world."*
7 The Enthusiast (Busy, fun-loving)	Seeks stimulation and pleasure Avoids pain and discomfort Wants to be free and independent	Rationalization: explains unacceptable thoughts, feelings and behaviors to themselves and others in a way that avoids their true motivation, intention, and the effects of their behavior *"It's not okay to feel/have pain, or to depend on others."*
8 The Challenger (Powerful, dominating)	Seeks control and justice Avoids feeling vulnerable or weak	Denial: unconsciously negates what makes them feel anxious by disavowing its very existence *"It's not okay to be vulnerable or to trust others in this unjust world."*
9 The Peacemaker (Easy-going, self-effacing)	Seeks harmony and comfort Avoids direct conflict and ill will	Narcotization: unconsciously numbs to avoid what feels too large, complex, difficult, or uncomfortable by engaging in prolonged rhythmic or routine activities that are familiar, require little attention, and provide comfort *"It's not okay to assert myself or rock the boat."*

In Lapid-Bogda's book, *Bringing Out the Best in Everyone You Coach*, she introduces the three levels of intelligence, stating, "Each of the nine Enneagram styles is rooted in one of the three centers, the head, the heart, or the body center. Although every person has all three centers of intelligence, each of us has a primary center, a secondary center, and a tertiary center. We rely on our primary center as a way of orienting to and experiencing the world."[7]

The head center helps us gather and process information, generate ideas, and plan. When it is not used in a positive way, an individual might struggle with analysis paralysis, anxiety, and over-planning, and fear may become the dominant emotion. The heart center helps us experience feelings and relate emotionally to others. When not used productively, the individual may struggle with emotional manipulation, oversensitivity, masking/playing roles, and depression, and sorrow may become the dominant feeling. The body is about action and inaction, physical sensations, and control. When not used appropriately, the person may tend toward over-activity or over-passivity, or become reactive or aggressive due to feeling out of control.

Our personalities give us areas of focus throughout our lives. Each Enneagram type views their environment through a unique lens that gives them a base to build on. The strength of heart types (Type 2, Type 3, and Type 4) lies in the emotional/spiritual dimension; the brain types (Type 5, Type 6, and Type 7) in the mind; and the body types (Type 8, Type 9, and Type 1) in the physical dimension.

We tend to choose partners and friends who have alternative areas of strength to ours. This allows our souls to learn about others despite the discomfort we feel about functioning from that perspective. As we expand from our base focus, we will learn to focus on other levels of intelligence (body, mind, and emotional/spiritual); this will support integration and strengthen our Creator Matrix.

In addition to the central personality type, each Enneagram type has two "wings" that can influence the personality. These are the types adjacent to the person's type. For example, a Type 3 like me will either be influenced by Type 2 or Type 4 traits. Usually, a person will lean more toward one than the other, particularly when they are under stress. This is all part of the bio-individuality of the personality.

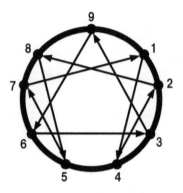

Finally, each number in the Enneagram diagram has an arrow pointing toward another number. Gurdjieff called this a "perpetual motion machine" and believed that personalities are always in motion. The arrows indicate which personality type you may default to when you're feeling insecure, fearful, or out of control—and, conversely, which personality type you may embody when you are operating as the most aligned version of yourself. For example, I have a friend who is a Type 5 with a 4 wing. When under stress, she tends to fall back into the erratic, ever-seeking patterns of the Type 7, which for her manifest as overspending, thrill-seeking, and constant feelings of "not having/doing/being enough." However, when at her best, she embodies the leadership qualities and impactful vision of the Type 8.

The Enneagram system has helped me understand myself more, including my strengths and weaknesses. It has also helped me in my relationships with other people. Understanding that my husband, Frans, as a Type 8, needs to feel "in control" helped me to accept the parts of his personality that are so different from my own. It also helped him understand that, as a Type 3, I care deeply about what people think and about achieving success. In fact, learning about the Enneagram also helped us understand why we are attracted to one another, and has brought more gratitude into our relationship. Frans helps me ground and learn how to hold boundaries. As a heart type, I am very emotional, and I have helped him to connect to his emotional side. Now that we understand our differences from an Enneagram point of view, we have more humor about things and become less irritated with each other.

Until we understand how important personality differences are and how they create a seamless unity among us as facets of Prime Creator, we will struggle with judgment and resistance to people who are different from us. However, when we have a basis for understanding different personality types, it's easier to stay curious instead of becoming reactive.

What I've presented is a very brief overview of the Enneagram and its potential for use as a self-discovery tool. However, even this basic information can become a launching point for your quest to uncover the beliefs at the root of your personality. A quick internet search will reveal any number of free Enneagram personality tests, as well as information, courses, and books to help you get started.

Other systems, like Human Design, DISC, Gene Keys, and others may also be of use in your pursuit of your bio-individual personality. However, it's important to remember that any personality typing system is only helpful insofar as it does not confine or limit your sense of self and your vision of what is possible for you to create; when that happens, the typing system has become just another unhelpful belief.

Beliefs, Emotions, and Stories are Intertwined

As we have learned in this chapter, our beliefs are intermingled with specific emotions and a particular life storyline. They are often stuck in the subconscious as a group because they are connected. Any aspect of them can be a triggering influence and can affect our life patterns and/or behavior. Consequently, these directly impact the storylines that consistently show up in our lives.

To truly change our lives and harness the power of our Creator Matrix, it is necessary to release limiting beliefs and low-frequency emotions that are often connected to our perception of ourselves and the world around us. We may need help with this process, and thankfully there are many great therapists and coaches available to support each person on their journey. In later chapters, I will explore various modalities that can address this.

It is important to remember that we are in a time of great change and acceleration, and that our ability to adapt quickly to these changes will determine how capable we become at navigating the consciousness of the new world.

Chapter Summary

- We are all unique. Our uniqueness influences our creativity, co-creations, and how we navigate certain situations we are in, choosing different paths influenced by our authentic nature.

- As human beings, we have beliefs about everything: ourselves, our health and wellness, our values, our worthiness, our abilities, our talents, our strengths and weaknesses, our families and communities, and the world as a whole and our place in it.

- Beliefs can be so strong that they amount to programming, underpinning, influencing, and controlling our self-talk and behavior and dominating our lives without us even knowing.

- Our beliefs are subjective and reflective of our relationship to our environment and the people around us (nurture, not nature); they are bio-individual aspects of our being that are unique and distinctive to us.

- Beliefs reside in the subconscious, and once embedded there they act as a programming tool for producing behavior patterns that are consistent with that belief.

- Beliefs don't need to remain static; we can change them and when we do, we can begin to change our lives.

- Limiting beliefs and low-frequency emotions stored in the subconscious are connected to undigested life experiences, fears, and traumas, and can hinder our full expression and self-actualization through our Creator Matrix.

- The subconscious can be reprogrammed with energy medicine and science-based therapies including EMDR, EFT, kinesiology, and Psych-K to release unhelpful beliefs, emotions, and storylines.

- Each of us has a unique personality that acts as a prism through which we view and experience our lives.

- When we know and accept ourselves, we can work with our personality. As we grow in consciousness, we become more understanding and accepting of how our personality affects ourselves and others.

Chapter Four

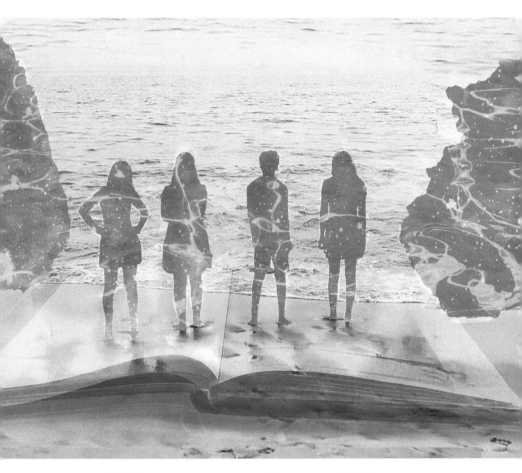

*Where in your Creator Matrix
is there a feeling of disconnection
and/or separation?*

"The measure of intelligence is the ability to change."

- Albert Einstein

CHAPTER FOUR

The Illusion of Separation and Disconnection

With all the changes unfolding in the galaxy and here on Earth, you'd think we would be rising into greater consciousness with ease, if not grace. However, the opposite seems to be true for many.

Our brains are programmed for survival. Therefore, we tend to perceive any change as threatening, and focus on the challenging or "bad" aspects of change rather than the good. Our brains are wired to see what we will lose from any change, not what we will gain. Change can also be frightening as we don't know exactly where it will lead to. Many people only focus on what is right before them and therefore fail to look beyond the obvious physical reality and the fact that we are connected to a great deal more. The real earthly illusion is that we are separate from each other and from a spiritual force or "higher power." In fact, science is now showing that we are all connected, and that the idea of a Universal Source may not be far-fetched after all.

During my holistic healing work, I came across people who already realized that they were connected to everything: the earth, the plants, the trees, the animals, and other people! These people can look beyond what is showing up on the physical level. By possessing this awareness, they are often better able to harness the power of these connections. They are connected and have integrated all areas of their Creator Matrix. Generally, these clients are more self-reflective, heal faster, and make changes with more ease. Ultimately, they are able to use their internal power to create the life they are looking for.

In contrast, other people seem completely unaware of these powerful connections and are more focused on the dimension of the physical. They tend not to believe in anything beyond what they can experience with their senses. There are also those who focus primarily on the spiritual/emotional and can't yet see the physical. Both of these experiences can leave the Creator Matrix unintegrated. I have learned in my healing work not to judge at what stage the client is but rather to meet the client where they are, realizing that every soul has their own path and tempo of evolution.

For example, at one spiritual retreat, our group meditated to the eighth dimension. On our break, I spoke to some of the participants and was struck by how many of them were physically ill and had manifested some sort of disease. It puzzled me that people who seemed so enlightened and connected spiritually could be so disconnected from their physical being—and, consequent to their physical health challenges, be unable to manifest what they truly desired here on Earth. They seemed physically drained and locked in a sort of perpetual searching mode.

Each soul functions in all dimensions at some level regardless of their conscious awareness. However, being too focused in one area can at times leave a person vulnerable and depleted in other areas. This can lead to feelings of disconnection and of being out of balance and can set the stage for the development of disease. Being focused primarily on one area for periods of time may be part of a normal evolutionary process, but when other areas are neglected completely, a susceptibility to imbalance can occur. This will be important as we begin to develop and integrate all areas of our Creator Matrix. As we grow in consciousness, we will ascend through different levels of awareness and integration. As we integrate, our soul will evolve, and we will learn to accept each perspective.

Disconnection

While working as a nurse, I was struck again and again by how many people were unaware of how sick they had become. They seemed disconnected on many levels—from their minds, bodies, and spirits. While caring for cancer patients, I was constantly surprised at how many had no idea how sick they really were. Before their diagnoses, many did not register any physical pain, discomfort, or symptoms beyond subtle cues like tiredness or minor aches and pains. However, many of them were suffering from some emotional crisis in their lives, like the loss of a loved one or a prolonged period of stress, which seemed to be the final straw.

Observing this inspired me to ask the question, "Could the disconnection these patients are experiencing have anything to do with their lack of wellness?"

This idea of disconnection plagued me for years, even after I stopped working as a nurse professionally. When answers came, it was through my own children's health challenges. Through my son, Frans Jr., I learned a great deal about the importance of a healthy immune system, and also the challenges many of us face to maintain healthy immunity with our modern lifestyle. Over the years, many of my clients have faced various health challenges because of a disconnection between what they were eating and their gut health, brain health, and the health of their immune system. Through my research, I have come to understand how closely related these three systems are to each other, and to the health of the whole.

My daughters taught me other lessons and broadened my awareness. My middle child, Kate, is curious, happy, and always had a tremendous excitement for life. However, from the time she could walk, she was constantly having accidents. It was so bad that, for a while, the local emergency room was asking my husband questions! She seemed to have no fear, and seemed not to realize that there are limitations here on Earth. For example, one day, I smelled the very familiar yet distinctive odor of my son's airplane glue. Turning to investigate, I saw my daughter's eyes glistening and shut. I instinctively knew that something was terribly wrong. I called our Dutch doctor, who, in a stern voice, instructed me to go immediately to the emergency room. When the ER doctor asked my daughter why she had glued her eyes shut, she responded, "To be beautiful." Yes, somehow my four-year-old had managed to climb ten shelves to reach the glue in order to make herself more beautiful. Luckily, the glue was removed and her eyes were fine—but this was just one of many incidents that showed me that she was not grounded or connected to earthly "rules." Only after many more years of these alarming experiences did I find a doctor who could help her connect to her physical body through exercises.

What does all this have to do with consciousness, intuition, and the Age of Aquarius? I promise, it will be clear in a moment.

You see, the more disconnected we are from our bodies, our cells, our emotions, our thoughts and thought forms, our belief systems, and our spiritual selves, the more disconnected we are from our whole-selves and the power of our Creator Matrix. This can throw us out of balance, which can lead to disease. The more disconnected we are, the less influence we are able to have on our own reality—including our wellness.

Our health is highly influenced and impacted by toxicity—whether that toxicity is physical, mental, or emotional. These areas are influenced by what we think, eat, the choices we make, and how we process our emotions. The actual word "disease" can be separated into two parts, "dis" and "ease," meaning "without ease or balance." Being well as a human has much to do with our ability to connect to all different aspects of ourselves. The more we grow in our consciousness, the more able we are to reflect on each of these different areas and take action to support them to become more integrated.

Resolving disconnection, like everything in life, requires a process of digestion, and the first step to digestion is awareness and allowance. When we pay attention to all areas of our lives, observe what we have allowed, and do what is necessary to bring ourselves back into balance, we are able to access greater levels of consciousness because more of our whole-self circuitry is online.

The second step, of course, is acceptance—of what has happened, what roles we played, and what stories we have created about those roles, and where we have been operating in the "shadow" aspects of our personalities. All of these must be accepted for us to resolve the disconnection, heal, and become whole. This is necessary not only to healing, but also in reaching the new version of ourselves as Creators.

The Wellness Wheel

During my nursing days, I had to sit with new patients, listen to their stories, take a history of what happened to them, take all their vital signs, and make an initial assessment of how serious their situation was. During these assessments, I was constantly evaluating where each individual patient was on the "illness-wellness continuum."

The Illness-Wellness Continuum was first proposed by John Travis in 1972. This concept draws a distinction between the "treatment paradigm" and the "wellness paradigm." The former runs from a neutral point without symptoms through progressions of signs, symptoms, disability, and premature death; while the latter runs across this spectrum and beyond the neutral point into conditions of awareness, education, growth, and high-level wellness.[1]

I've adapted this concept in the graphic below.

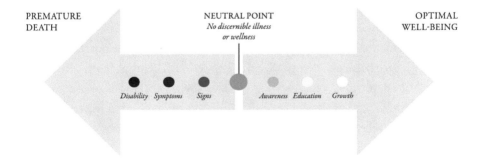

PREMATURE DEATH · NEUTRAL POINT *No discernible illness or wellness* · OPTIMAL WELL-BEING

Disability Symptoms Signs   *Awareness Education Growth*

We all exist somewhere on this continuum, and our daily choices and life stories propel us to move along this scale in either direction. Obviously, when we become sick, we gravitate toward the "signs and symptoms" side of the scale; when we are well, we move toward the "wellness" direction. Over the years, I realized that each person's starting place was different—and, therefore, so was the place where they could possibly end up on the spectrum. Some leaned toward becoming increasingly ill, while others used their experience as a "wake-up call" to make major changes in their lives and advance toward wellness.

The problem I saw was that our hospitals were geared to an illness-based system and had very little time to help patients resolve disconnections and make the changes necessary to create true wellness. Instead, the system sought to take people at the "illness" end of the spectrum and return them to a more neutral place. However, if everyone exists somewhere between illness and wellness, being without illness does not necessarily mean that one is "well." In fact, if one is simply "not ill," one is existing in the middle of the continuum, not at its positive extreme.

This really bothered me. It seemed like only people with enough wealth and a high level of consciousness—meaning, they were able to perceive the disconnection they were experiencing and take proactive steps to resolve it—could get the help they needed to achieve lasting change toward wellness and avert the crisis of complete dis-balance and disease. Most of the people I saw in the hospital were merely surviving; the concept of thriving did not even exist for them. Their desired outcome was to return to that neutral zone of "not ill."

One key attribute of health coaching is that we are not satisfied with the absence of disease. We strive to see our clients progress toward the best possible versions of themselves, with optimal health at the "wellness" end of the continuum. This is possible for all of us—even if we have received a challenging diagnosis or have had issues with disconnection in the past.

Travis further explores a multidimensional concept of wellness using the analogy of the "Wellness Wheel," where he looks at the many areas of a person's life that can influence their wellness trajectory. These include: self-responsibility/love; breathing; sensing; eating; moving; feeling; thinking; playing/working; communicating; intimacy; finding meaning; and transcending.[(2)] Using the assessment wheel enables a person to become aware of areas in which they may currently be experiencing disconnection, areas that might be lacking in fulfillment, and areas that require personal development and change.

When "wellness" is centered around a holistic vision of body, mind, and spirit, consciousness becomes the most potent medicine. As we grow in our awareness, we make choices about which areas we wish to develop. Depending on our stories, beliefs, and personality type, we may be hyper-focused on one area, to the detriment of others. Developing the capacity to observe this, expand our awareness, and allow more light/information to enter our bodies will always support our efforts in the direction of wellness.

Moreover, as we explore the concept of energy in Chapter Six, we will learn that the dominant energy in our bio-individual electromagnetic field influences what energies are brought through into our reality as matter. In other words, what we focus on expands. My clients who are able to focus on wellness with all their senses, including what that would mean and feel like for them, often improve their health. I know many examples of people who, through the power of their mind and trust in a higher power, went into complete remission from cancer. Even those who were not able to overcome their illness were able to heal aspects of their being before leaving the Earthly plane.

Ultimately, we will bring more health, healing, and wellness into our reality as we focus on it, as we desire it, and as we are inspired by it. When we are constantly focusing on preventing illness, we are still holding the consciousness and frequency of the word "illness." In order to shift this, we need to shift our perspective to focus on wellness and what brings us closer to it.

Why is the illness-wellness continuum important for our purposes here? Because it's also a continuum of consciousness and connection! When we consciously observe, connect to, and learn to work with our bio-individual electromagnetic field, we can use our power as Creators to influence our experience of health. The more connected we are to our energy, and the more we can clear our energy channels of undigested stories and emotions, the healthier we will become on all levels!

However, there is one factor that, no matter how conscious we become, can undermine our ability to manage and direct our energy consciously—and that factor is stress.

What is Stress, and How Does it Affect Us?

Our brain functions much like a computer that stores and processes data and information. With too much data input, a computer will become overwhelmed and crash. Our brain functions in much the same way. When we are overloaded, our bodily systems can "short-circuit," leading to burnout.

If the brain is the "hardware" of the body, our thoughts, emotions, DNA, and stored memories are the software. When the pressures of life exceed our ability to cope, our body gives us signals. For example, when we are unable to process more sensory or informational input, we might suffer from headaches, muscle tension, anxiety, panic, brain fog, inability to focus, depression, heart palpitations, chest pain, anger or rage, fatigue, social isolation, substance abuse, lack of motivation, loss of spiritual connection and purpose, and sleep issues, to name just a few.

When many of us reach this point of system overload, we say, "I'm stressed out!"

The Farlex Free Medical Dictionary defines stress as, "An organism's total response to environmental demands or pressures ... Stress in humans results from interactions between persons and their environment that are perceived as straining or exceeding their adaptive capacities and threatening their well-being."[3] Our ancient cave-dwelling ancestors lived their lives by hunting and gathering and faced literal life and death challenges on a daily basis. Today many of us experience stress yet are not facing literal life or death challenges. The problem lies within our biological system's response. When we get a feeling that we are in danger, whether real or imagined, the physiological response is the same.

Stress is something all of us must contend with. The speed of our modern-day life can exacerbate the amount of pressure that we feel each and every day. This in turn influences the health and well-being of our bodies, minds, and spirits. However, most of us don't really understand stress until we experience its negative effects for ourselves.

On the one hand, stress is necessary for inspiration, excitement, and purpose. When we are facing a deadline or meeting a challenge, we can attain new heights of focus, drive, and stamina. However, when stress is prolonged, it can take over and, without us even noticing, cause debilitating reactions to our entire being.

Stress has a direct effect on our hormonal system. The amygdala—the part of our brain responsible for our instinctual and survival-related behaviors—is stimulated when we have challenges, our safety is threatened, or we sense a degree of danger. In response, our body sends out a cascade of hormonal reactions that help us cope by fighting, fleeing, or freezing.

The "fight, flight, or freeze" response stimulates the production of cortisol, which in turn stimulates our adrenal glands. Cortisol is a naturally occurring steroid hormone activated by the hypothalamic-pituitary-adrenal (HPA) axis. When cortisol is released, sugar is also released into the bloodstream to ensure a person has the energy to run quickly. Blood and energy are sent to our arms and legs to allow us to run away or react with speed and urgency. This response has a consequence for the rest of our body because blood and energy are diverted from our brain and gut—the places where reasoning, emotional processing, and digestion happen.

Think of it as a built-in fire alarm for the body. In small doses, cortisol can have many positive effects, like keeping us motivated and focused, supporting our immune system by keeping inflammation low, helping to control our sleep/wake cycle, and helping us maintain overall balance within our body's systems. However, too much of a good thing can also have detrimental effects. Imagine living with a fire alarm going off in the background all the time! You wouldn't be able to relax! Cortisol overload produces much the same effect.

When we have too much cortisol in our systems, we can lose our connection to our intuition, logic, and reason. Just think about how people you know act when they are under stress. They might come across as entirely different from who they normally are. They might stop thinking logically and calmly, and instead become overly reactive, nervous, panicked, or angry; in some cases, this can lead to violence, while in others it can lead to anxiety, panic attacks, or even self-harm. Now, think further about some of our modern-day problems and conflicts. How much of what we are experiencing is a direct result of our systems being overloaded?

Long-term stress can also contribute to overeating and obesity as our body attempts to make up for its excessive sugar usage. The original problem was caused by too much cortisol. Once the body signals the alarm, cortisol is released and the reaction is either fight, flight, or freeze. Cortisol stimulates the liver to release more and more sugar into the bloodstream (from glycogen), thus raising blood sugar levels. Furthermore, it stimulates the pancreas to release more insulin as well, and this then triggers a hunger response. If this cycle of chronic stress continues, then the person involved (who is often simply sitting behind their desk or in a car) will not use the sugar and it will be stored in the body as fat—and, in particular, as abdominal fat, which accumulates around and between the vital organs. Over time, this chronic stress causes the pancreas to become increasingly depleted, which raises the incidence of insulin resistance and diabetes.

Over time, chronic stress may affect many other aspects of our health and well-being. Today, we are seeing an epidemic of people developing a cluster of health conditions called metabolic syndrome. This syndrome occurs when an individual has developed three of the following five conditions: high blood glucose, low HDL cholesterol, high triglycerides, large waist circumference, and/or high blood pressure.[4] If a person is overweight, for example, has high blood pressure, and is under a great deal of stress, they are far more vulnerable to developing high blood sugar.

Similarly, if a person with diabetes and excessive stress may, over time, develop high blood pressure. Once a person has metabolic syndrome, they are more at risk of developing diabetes, heart disease, and stroke.

The chronic spiking of blood sugar has been linked to what many now call Type 3 diabetes. Our brain and gut are interconnected, and an inflamed gut is often mirrored in our brain. Inflammation in the brain can contribute to the development of Alzheimer's disease or dementia. Science is also showing that people in a chronic state of stress are more prone to immune/digestion system dysfunction, cancer, mental health issues, as well as all kinds of relationship issues and career challenges.

In general, people are not the best versions of themselves when they are in a prolonged state of stress. Over time, operating in the state of "not their best selves"—aka, survival mode—can leave people even more disconnected from their body, mind, and spirit complex.

STRESS AND DISCONNECTION

How does stress lead to disconnection on the body, mind, and spirit level?

On the physical level, when we are in a constant state of flight or fight, we don't have time to rest, digest, or repair, which means that we don't have time to eliminate toxins from the body. This eventually leads to a breakdown in cellular function and chronic inflammation. This chronic inflammation causes a disconnection at the cell level— particularly at a cell-to-cell communication level. Our cells simply cannot function well if they are overloaded with toxins. Many people who are under chronic stress also experience sleep problems. During sleep, we detox our physical body as well as our mental and emotional bodies. On a mental level, when we don't detox our minds, our neurons can become disconnected and chaotic. We can experience memory and concentration issues. On an emotional level, when we don't have time to rest and digest, we are unable to process our emotions. These blocked emotions also cause disconnection at the cellular level. And finally, when the entire system is continuously blocked, it will affect the ability of our whole body, mind, and spirit complex to work together as a unified field as well as within the unified field. How can we expect to create what we desire from such a place?

MANAGING STRESS

Learning how to manage stress is one of the most important areas of self-care. Physically, humans can manage stress and mitigate its negative effects by creating balance between the sympathetic and parasympathetic nervous systems. The sympathetic nervous system is responsible for the "fight, flight, or freeze" response, while the parasympathetic system is responsible for a "rest and digest" response. We need them both, and therefore we need to learn to manage both.

According to a recent study entitled "Chronic Stress, Cortisol Dysfunction, and Pain: A Psychoneuroendocrine Rationale for Stress Management in Pain Rehabilitation," the sympathetic nervous system promotes catabolic tissue breakdown and fat metabolism to mobilize glucose for energy, arousal, alertness, motivation, and goal-directed behavior. At the other end of the spectrum, the parasympathetic nervous system promotes healing, repair, immunity, and the anabolic growth required for restored energy reserves and longevity."[5]

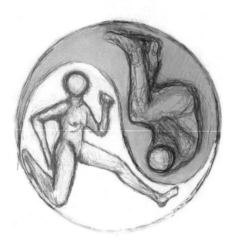

How we learn to balance our sympathetic and parasympathetic systems has much to do with how well we care for ourselves. Poor lifestyle habits combined with too much cortisol from stress can ultimately repress immune system function and negatively influence the health of the gut. When there is not enough time and space to "rest and digest," the result can be poor digestion and inflammation on a physical level, which is the basis for most illnesses. On a mental and spiritual level, it can mean undigested emotions and unhelpful stories, which contribute to energetic blockages. When the stress is intense, it creates trauma, which impacts the system on all levels. This is why learning to manage our stress is one of the most important areas of self-care.

There are healthy levels of stress that motivate performance and drive away boredom and apathy, and there are unhealthy levels of chronic stress that produce disease. Humanity cannot move forward into a new, more peaceful world without cleansing harmful past stress and turning off the flight-or-fight response. We need to create safety within ourselves, including through learning and using stress management techniques. We can move beyond the mere survival mode and knee-jerk reaction patterns to emotional freedom. We are here not to survive, but to feel alive and to thrive to our fullest. The New Earth we are ascending toward is about thriving, not just getting by.

As discussed in Chapter Two, as Creators our energy can move outward (yang), or inward (yin). All human beings are comfortable with a combination of these two energetic principles. Some love to be out in the world trying new things, while others prefer staying quiet, observing, and digesting. The truth is, we need both to create a balanced life. When we have an excess of either yin or yang, stress can result. However, as we are all uniquely co-creating our lives, our "optimal" balance of energy will look different from those around us, and will also change during different periods of our lives.

Stress can be acute when we experience a major event, like a death in the family, a financial crisis, loss of employment, divorce, or sudden illness. When stress comes upon us suddenly, it's easy to recognize that we have become stressed. However, stress can also be chronic, meaning it can build up slowly over time to debilitating levels. When this happens, a person may be totally unaware that they are in trouble. How well we handle stress depends a great deal on how well we have learned to care for ourselves. Handling chronic stress has more to do with how we manage our inner balance over a long period of time.

When a computer gets overloaded, we can be proactive by cleaning our hard drive and running certain programs to avert a crash. In much the same way, we as humans can preventively take steps to manage our stress levels.

The first (and possibly most important) step in self-care is learning to reflect on the need for it. Once we become conscious of how much we have taken in from the outside world, we can begin to recognize our need to digest and release excess energy in the form of thoughts, emotions, and experiences. As the American philosopher and psychologist William James wrote, "The greatest weapon against stress is our ability to choose one thought over another." As you now understand, we have a choice in what we think about, both consciously and subconsciously; we can choose how we think about stress, too.

The second step is to address the effects that stress has had on our levels of body, mind, and spirit. As mentioned above, excess stress has a direct effect on multiple bodily systems. When left unchecked, it can cause burnout. When we are physically near burnout, we are often mentally challenged as well, experiencing such symptoms as depression, anxiety, or panic disorders. Spiritually, we can become disconnected from our unique, authentic selves. We can feel alone, abandoned, and confused about where we are going. We can also disconnect from both Source energy and grounding energy from the earth. This can affect the health of our meridians and chakra centers, causing energetic stagnancy or blockages.

The final step is, of course, to learn how to manage stress. Thankfully, there are many ways to manage stress nowadays. As we are all unique, we can choose which options suit us best. Many people choose to seek preventative integrative treatments like acupuncture, Ayurveda, neurofeedback therapy, family constellation therapy, osteopathy, kinesiology, orthomolecular therapy, classic homeopathy, reflexology, massage, energy healing, reiki, color therapy, and aromatherapy to remain in balance energetically and physically. Developing healthy lifestyle habits such as regular exercise, breathing and relaxation techniques, mindfulness, yoga, good nutrition, and walking in nature, to name just a few, is vital for many. Others find listening to music, painting, or writing to be therapeutic stress relievers. As I mentioned earlier, my self-care journey began when I learned to meditate. While this was a relatively unknown modality when I began, today it is considered a well-established practice to help rebalance the body, mind, and spirit. You can find all sorts of meditation apps, health coaches, personal trainers, and nutritional apps to help support and guide you on your health journey. Looking at all aspects of our lifestyle choices is essential when making these changes.

Healing and Integrating our Dualistic Aspects

For eons, we have navigated our relationship with our life stories through a dualistic perspective. Duality is "the quality or state of having two different or opposite parts or elements."[6] This has a direct effect on how we look at our lives and experience ourselves as Creators.

In some ways, duality can be helpful. Living on Earth has been a unique opportunity for each of us to experience what duality feels like. We learn about light through understanding the dark, love through understanding hate, and joy through understanding sadness. The inverse is also true: we learn about dark through light, hate through love, and sadness through joy. When we can see life from different viewpoints, we can have more compassion and understanding for each experience and each other.

However, as we grow in consciousness, we are being asked to integrate the dark and light into a unified whole. The new moon looks dark, the full moon looks white—but it is all just the moon. So it is with our quantum reality: all things are present at the same time and exist simultaneously.

Duality isn't a challenge for us as Creators when we can hold both viewpoints simultaneously. However, the process of observing separate viewpoints without maintaining the awareness of wholeness can result in a feeling of separation, rather than connectedness. Remaining in duality can result in disconnection on all levels of body, mind, and/ or spirit. This disconnection can be the cause for us to rely on negative habits for coping, developing health challenges, discordant relationships, and overall disempowered ways of being. When we can hold both perspectives in a duality without judgment, we will come to a point where we no longer need to experience opposition in order to grow and change. We will no longer need to experience hate to know love, or dark to know light. We will simply integrate our understanding of the desired state and "become it."

Reaching the "become it" stage can be challenging. Most of the time, when uncomfortable feelings arise or we are confronted with cognitive dissonance, we are not able to completely digest and work through it on our own. As we'll explore in more depth in upcoming chapters, we even collect memories in our cellular structures—from our adult lives, our childhoods, and even from our ancestors. These can create blockages in both the body and the energy field at the cellular level.

Many healers help people to integrate these disconnected parts of themselves, which are a result of wounds they carry on all levels of body, mind, and spirit. If these wounds go unhealed, we continue to neglect these blocked parts of ourselves. When these wounded aspects come from childhood trauma or other life-altering experiences, it may be necessary to work to identify and release them with a qualified therapist. These traumas can occur on all levels of body, mind, and spirit, and are bio-individual because our perceptions are different. A trauma can be more impactful if it is also carried through our familial DNA, or from other incarnations. Traumas can cause disconnection ("splitting of the soul") by their very nature. Whatever the chosen healing pathway, addressing and reconciling the duality in our experience helps us to both release the trauma from our Creator Matrix and simultaneously integrate its meaning for us. When we do this, our body, mind, spirit matrix will become more coherent and reconnected.

Many refer to this integrative work as "shadow work." We all have a "shadow side" that has been hidden and/or neglected. It takes a great deal of courage to see and address this shadow side, in the same way it takes courage to navigate the dark when we are used to the light. The exposure of the darker side of both ourselves and humanity can be frightening—mostly because we have judged and avoided it instead of integrating and accepting it.

We can compare shadow work to the act of peeling an onion. When we peel an onion, we can peel it layer by layer. If we visualize each layer having its own unique storyline, we begin the shadow work by releasing one layer at a time. We understand that the blockages of each layer are somehow connected to the layer beneath, as well as to the core or center. Each layer reveals a more in-depth view of the storyline and blockage. When we peel an onion, our eyes start to water, and we may want to step away; so, too, can shadow work be an uncomfortable process. Through shadow work, we make the unconscious conscious, release the block-ages, and eventually become united with our core self.

One day, when I was under hypnosis, I connected to one of my past lives. The vision seemed very real; more important, however, were the emotions that came up.

In that lifetime, I was a scientist. In my vision, I saw myself doing all kinds of experiments on other humans in the name of science and prog-ress. The worst part, though, was the complete separation I felt from any emotions related to what I was doing and had done to others. In my "afterlife review" of that life, I recall being unable to accept myself and forgive myself for the pain I had caused.

In duality, our souls come in willing to play all sides of the story. Some of us play the victim, others the perpetrator, and still others the savior. We eventually play all the different roles so we can learn to understand all aspects of duality and/or opposition.

Some of us prefer playing one role and judge the others. For instance, it is easier to feel compassion for the victim, paint the rescuer as a hero, and hate the perpetrator of a story.

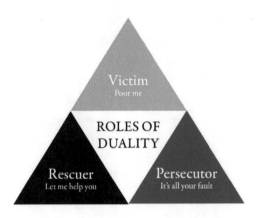

What helped me rise above the judgments of duality was to realize how lonely it must be to play the perpetrator. The illusion of playing out these roles is that we *are* these roles. That is when we become stuck. We can experience the different parts vicariously through watching movies or listening to the stories of others. In our awakening, we are tasked to develop compassion for everyone and for each role. It is time for all of us to heal, integrate and rise above both the roles and the stories. Then and only then can we heal and allow our Creator Matrix to become united and whole.

Many of us, in our process of reintegrating, will remember experiences, traumas, stories in family lines, and even past life stories. I have found in my healing work with clients that it is not necessary to remember all the stories to heal, only the ones that have caused an extreme block or repeating storyline. For example, my vision of remembering the past life I have shared above has helped me see and identify the root cause of my fear around hurting others. Even as a child, I was unconsciously avoiding a part of myself, and this avoidance manifested as a crippling fear. To step more fully into my power as the Creator, I had to accept that a part of me had hurt somebody else (intentionally or unintentionally) and forgive that part of me. Only then could I become more integrated and healed.

The gift of moving beyond duality is that I am now able to love myself more fully. Moreover, I am able to see others with love, despite any roles they have played, and therefore help them love themselves. I now realize that each of us are heroes for being willing to come here on Earth to play these roles for the benefit of each other and the process of experiencing who we are.

Shadow work is not simply going back in time to relive past stories and figure out the "why" of our disconnections, habits, and behaviors. For many, that can be not only unhelpful, but can actually reinforce feelings of separateness and dualistic perspectives. Instead, it's about looking at the stories and releasing the emotional charges, judgments, and fears associated with them. Again, we are not our stories. We have experienced and participated in stories for the benefit of our evolution—but the time has come to reintegrate our disconnected Creator Matrix and move beyond duality into unity. As part of that journey, we must accept and offer love to all parts of ourselves, even the "dark" sides. Only then can we digest and integrate these aspects of our being to become whole.

It all begins with self-observation and the decision to make changes. Many start their healing journey by doing this deep shadow work, while others start by improving different aspects of their lifestyle. It does not matter where you begin, only that you decide to begin. I have observed that each soul will eventually want to expand and move forward in all areas of healing, as energy seeks resolution and expansion.

Lifestyle Choices: Choosing to Change

If there is an overarching theme to this book, it's this: we have a choice, and we can change. Science indicates that lifestyle choices play a role in all areas of our health and wellness. Choosing to change parts of our lifestyle requires that *we* decide to change.

When I say "lifestyle choices," I don't just mean food and exercise, but all areas of the Wellness Wheel that we consciously engage and interact with. Remember our discussion in Chapter Two about primary and secondary food? Well, your primary food is the *energy* that you feed into all areas of your life.

Understanding how thoughts, beliefs, story, and energy work, and how we create from our energy field, helps us to understand how we can change. This science is teaching us that through observation and intention, we can make new neural connections that help us to make these changes and make them last. If we want to change, we must change the vibration of our bio-individual electromagnetic field by creating new thoughts, beliefs, and feelings that support the change we are looking for. This process will create new neural pathways in our brain, and over time, these changes will become part of who we are. However, we must first observe the need and desire for this change.

Life is about more than just survival. Many people spend their whole lives in survival mode, but this is not ideal for us as Creators. As we realize the power of our Creator Matrix, we learn that how we think and feel truly matters, and that the best way to get out of survival mode is to truly believe that life is not about survival. Making intentions and reprogramming our subconscious is a powerful tool in starting to change this limiting belief. When working with clients, I often have them add "life is easy for me" to their intentions.

Changing bad habits into good is recognized as one of the most effective ways to improve health and wellness. But, as with many aspects of our evolution, it is easier said than done. Stacks of books have been written on how to change habits. They cover a range of topics, from threatening addictions like alcoholism, emotional eating, and gambling, to relationship improvements like just being nice to others. Many authors agree that making small but consistent alterations on a daily basis and sticking to them is the key to amazing medium- and long-term results. However, sticking to them with persistence is the tricky part.

Habits help us cope with our experiences and life itself. Habits serve us until they don't. We usually only recognize that they no longer serve us once they make us feel uncomfortable and/or hurt us. Habits can affect us negatively, contributing to our disconnection on all levels of body, mind, and spirit over time. When we are disconnected, we are not connected to the emotional and physical signals our bodies are sending us. However, while they might help us ignore or reduce the intensity of stress in the moment, some habits can keep us from accessing and becoming conscious of the very stories and energies that are keeping us stuck.

We explored this a bit in Chapter Two, when we learned how our habits are born from and related to our stories. Now, we'll look at habits from a different angle: neuroplasticity.

Neuroplasticity tells us that the more we repeat a particular action or thought pattern, the more embedded it becomes, until the point at which the behavior has become automatic. Repeating something consistently over time creates a habit. The longer this is done, the more this "habit" becomes embedded in the brain, and the more resistant we can become to changing this behavior. The concept is simple: the more flexible we are, the easier it is to change. The more rigid we are, the more difficult it is for us to change. The more neuroplasticity the brain has, the more flexible and adaptive it is to learning new ways and making new neural pathways. Disconnection at the cellular level can occur as our neuroplasticity decreases.

Here's a good example of this. When you're driving home from work or shopping, the car sometimes seems to guide itself home on automatic pilot. You can walk from the bed to your toilet in the middle of the night when you're half asleep. But what happens when you move to another home? How long does it take for that automatic behavior pattern to develop again? The experts disagree: some say twenty-one days, others twenty-eight, others two months or more. The more important factor is not how long it takes, but how many repetitions of the behavior are made. The more repetitions, the faster the learning. Some people may be triggered to change by a shocking life event, like a health crisis. We often refer to this as a "wake-up call." Others may be triggered to change at different points in their life as they become more conscious and aware of how their habits are serving (or not serving) their highest well-being.

Change can be difficult, or it can be easy. It can happen quickly, or it can take time. In the end, it's up to you. When assessing how you want to create change, it can be helpful to reflect on how you've handled change in the past, especially change that you didn't choose or ask for. Just like all habits have their stories, we all have our stories around change. But, like all stories, these can be rewritten to reflect what you desire as the Creator of your life.

Now, consider how disconnection and habits work together.

If your habits are facilitating disconnection in any area of your life, what needs to be addressed first? Your habits, or the disconnection?

For better or worse, it's your habits.

The truth is, if changing habits were easy, everyone would be effortlessly leading healthy, happy lives. However, particularly for those dealing with stress and/or disconnection, change can feel almost impossible, because there are many factors beyond the habits that need to be resolved. If you are experiencing disconnection, you may be using your habits to actively avoid facing something in your life. However, by working on your habits and lifestyle choices, you can open the door to conscious observation of the disconnection and begin to apply your awareness to find a path toward digestion and integration.

THE SCIENCE OF CHANGE

We live in a world where we are constantly interacting with others. This process is called co-creation.

As we interact with others, we are influenced by their energy fields, personalities, belief systems, emotions, conflicts, physical presence, and stories. Learning how to react to all of these variables with wisdom, maturity, and unconditional love will make us co-creative masters.

Sometimes in our life stories, we can feel changes are imposed. For example, as a child, I did not choose for my family to move every couple of years, and I was sad to leave the friends I had made. However, even though the change was destabilizing, I also learned to enjoy the excitement of new towns and cities, new friendships, and new experiences, and therefore learned to become more flexible and adaptive in the process.

How we deal with change is personal and subjective. Some crave it, while others fear it. Some feel both ways at the same time. In order to understand our complex relationship with change, we need to look at cognitive dissonance and the role it plays in the change story.

We learned about the role of cognitive dissonance with regard to belief systems in Chapter Three. Now, let's look at it in terms of life-style change.

Cognitive dissonance is part of the "change story." Making a change requires a decision to do so. This initial decision requires that our old beliefs and habits become uncomfortable enough that we are willing to change them. As we have learned, we have certain beliefs that govern our behavior and choices. When new information comes in and contradicts these old beliefs and ideas, we may experience cognitive dissonance.

Assimilating new information can be confusing and uncomfortable. Our logical or "left" brain adopts beliefs that serve our habits and relates to incoming information based on those beliefs. The creative or "right" side of the brain, however, is creative, curious, and constantly encourages us to grow and change by thinking outside the box. Therefore, when new information comes in, it can be uncomfortable, as our two "modes" of relating to information seem to clash. If our creative and change-oriented brain wins this argument, we may change our beliefs to accommodate this new information. However, if our logical brain prevails, we may deny the new information altogether because it "doesn't make sense" according to our current belief systems.

According to the Stages of Change Model developed by researchers James Prochaska and Carlo DiClemente, there are six stages of change: pre-contemplation, contemplation, determination, action, mainte-nance, and termination. As people move through these stages, they get closer to adopting a new habit or behavior. By recognizing where you are in the change process, you can reflect on what is needed to move to the next stage. The goal of any change process is to move through the stages to reach the "maintenance" level, where the behavior is so auto-matic that it feels natural. Only then can "termination" be attained, where the new behavior is integrated so completely that there is little chance of recidivism.

Here is a more complete breakdown of the Stages of Change Model.[7]

1. **Pre-contemplation:** In this stage, we do not intend to take action to change in the foreseeable future (meaning, within six months). We may be unaware that our behavior is problematic or that it creates negative effects for us or others. We may also be thinking of reasons not to change our behavior and arguing for its continuance.

2. **Contemplation:** In this stage, we come to a point of intending to start a new behavior in the near future (within six months). We recognize that our current behavior is no longer serving us and that a different behavior may be healthier or more helpful. We begin to weigh the pros and cons of changing and may feel that there are equal benefits and risks to the change we are considering.

3. **Determination:** In this stage, we are ready to take action on our plan for change within thirty days. We may take small steps toward the change, because we recognize that this change will improve something about our lives.

4. **Action:** In this stage, we have changed our behavior and intend to keep acting and making decisions in alignment with that change.

5. **Maintenance:** In this stage, we have sustained our behavior change for more than six months and are working to prevent ourselves from "relapsing" into earlier change stages. The new behavior is beginning to feel natural and requires less effort at this stage.

6. **Termination.** In this stage, we have lost the desire to return to our old behavior and are sure we will not do so. We have successfully created a new way of being.

Stages of Change Model

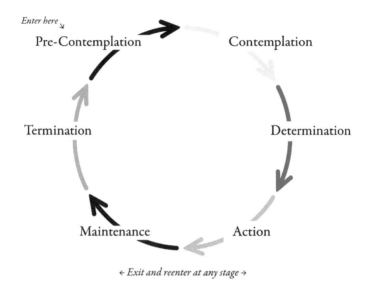

← Exit and reenter at any stage →

We are not trapped by our habits. We can choose them—and, by moving through the Cycles of Change, allow them to become part of who we are. When old habits stop serving us, cognitive dissonance and feelings of discomfort will increase; this is often what pushes us from the Pre-contemplation to the Contemplation stage.

As we change our habits, our frequency changes, too. When we move away from lifestyle choices that do not serve our optimal well-being, we will experience greater clarity and capacity both in our physical body and in our energy field.

The opposite is also true: as our frequency changes, so too do our habits. When we are under stress or have experienced trauma, we may revert to old habits, or develop new, unhealthy habits to cope with our current situation. When we experience an "upleveling" in consciousness, old habits may no longer feel right for us. As in all things, our ability to consciously observe our thoughts, beliefs, and stories will serve us well here.

In the next chapter, we will look more deeply at what consciousness is, and how understanding it can improve our life's purpose and overall well-being.

Chapter Summary

- The real earthly illusion is that we are separate from each other and from a spiritual force or "higher power." In fact, science is showing that we are all connected, and that the idea of a Universal Source may not be far-fetched after all.

- The more disconnected we are from our bodies, cells, emotions, thoughts, thought forms, belief systems, and spiritual selves, the more we become disconnected from our whole selves and the power of our Creator Matrix, and the less influence we are able to have on our own reality, including our wellness.

- Our health is highly influenced and impacted by physical, mental, and emotional toxicity, which is influenced by what we think, the choices we make, and how we process emotions.

- Awareness, allowance, and acceptance of what happened, what roles we played, and what stories we have created about it are necessary to resolve disconnection, healing, and reaching the new versions of ourselves as Creators. Only then can we allow our Creator Matrix to become united and whole.

- In health coaching, we are not satisfied with the absence of disease and merely surviving, we strive to see clients progress toward the best possible versions of themselves, with optimal health at the "wellness" end of the "Illness-Wellness Continuum", the concept of thriving.

- Stress is a result of information overload and affects us on all levels of body, mind, and spirit. Some stress is necessary for inspiration, excitement, and purpose, and is good for our well-being, mental health, and behavior.

- Our stress system is designed for survival. Through a series of hormonal reactions to feeling unsafe, the body will try to protect itself by entering into a "fight or flight" response— or in some cases, a 'freeze' response.

- As a result, prolonged, chronic stress can have debilitating reactions on our entire being at all levels—body, mind, and spirit. This can lead to a person feeling overly reactive, nervous, panicked, angry, and anxious; and possibly developing habits like emotional eating.

- Learning to manage our stress is one of the most important areas of self-care. Physically humans can manage stress and mitigate its negative effects by creating balance between the sympathetic ("fight, flight, or freeze" response—promoting arousal, alertness, motivation, and goal-directed behavior) and parasympathetic ("rest and digest"—promoting healing, repair, immunity, restoring energy reserves, and longevity) nervous systems.

- Duality has given us the opportunity to experience what each of the dualistic sides feels like (light/dark, love/hate, joy/sadness). As we grow in consciousness, we are asked to integrate dark and light into a unified whole, moving beyond duality into unity.

- Shadow work involves healing disconnected aspects of our Creator Matrix. This can involve healing traumas that have occurred in childhood or traumas that have been life altering. Through shadow work we make the unconscious conscious, release blockages, and eventually become united with our core self.

- Learning how to interact with others with wisdom, maturity, and unconditional love will make us co-creative masters.

- When we begin to change our thoughts, beliefs, feelings, and habits we can begin the process of change. The Stages of Change Model is based on the concept that people need time to change their behaviors and that change occurs in six stages: Pre-contemplation, Contemplation, Preparation, Action, Maintenance, and Termination.

- We are not trapped by our habits; we can choose them. By changing our habits, our frequency changes too. By moving away from lifestyle choices that don't serve our optimal well-being, we will experience greater clarity and capacity in both our physical body and in our energy field.

Chapter Five

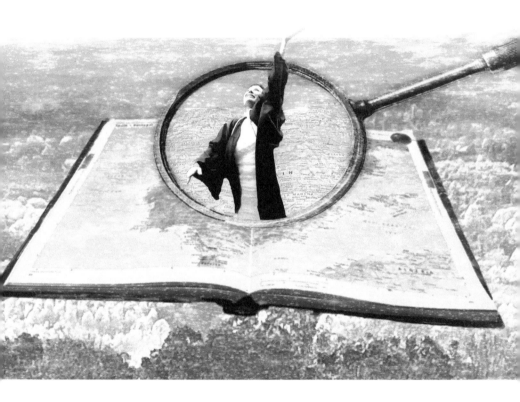

What you focus on expands.
Where are you putting your attention?

"The key to growth is the introduction of higher dimensions of consciousness into our awareness."

- Lao Tzu

CHAPTER FIVE

Consciousness

A few times thus far in this book, we've mentioned "consciousness" and "becoming conscious." But what does that mean, exactly? What is consciousness, and why is it something we should pursue?

Consciousness is an all-encompassing word that I believe has a strong connection to why we are here. Many spiritual masters are helping us now to understand consciousness. Although many find it difficult to describe exactly, to me, consciousness is the state of knowing oneself or "knowingness" in general. It begins with our perceptions and ability to observe ourselves, others, and all that is in our awareness.

In order to claim our power as Creators, we must first become conscious. Synonyms for this state of being might include: recognition, awareness, attentiveness, mindfulness, understanding, enlightenment, and alertness—although in practice these are just a fraction of what consciousness entails.

In my experience, when people start expanding their consciousness, they ask important questions like, "Who am I?" and "Why have I arrived on Planet Earth?" I seemed to be doing this from quite a young age. In fact, as I was asking this question and searching for answers, at that time it seemed very few people around me were asking this at all. This left me feeling lonely and confused. However, once I asked these key questions, I never stopped asking them; rather, each discovery left me even more curious. It came up repeatedly at crisis points in my life when I was unsure in which direction I should go.

These days, I am amazed by how many people have not yet reached the point of asking these questions. Once you ask them, growing in consciousness becomes an inevitable next step.

So, what exactly is consciousness, and what can we become conscious of? Science is showing us that the base for consciousness is energy. When we look at consciousness as energy, we have the opportunity to become aware of everything that exists at all levels of life, including the physical, mental, emotional, and spiritual planes of existence. Put more simply, consciousness is life force—the force that allows all creation to exist. Imagine that the life force is the force that steers the car and chooses the path the car will go.

When people begin to awaken, they develop the capacity to look beyond the illusion of the physical and focus on other dimensions of reality simultaneously. They realize that we are not physical beings having a spiritual experience, but rather spiritual beings having a physical experience. This is a major jump in consciousness! We see through the illusion of separation and begin to realize that we are part of a far larger field which connects us all. At this point, we can look beyond our physical reality for answers and shift our focus from the external, materialistic world to our internal world of self-development and self-realization. We can then become aware of the parts of us we have denied and ignored, and look for answers and healing in the dimensions of mind, emotion, and spirit.

Several years ago, I began writing down the words "The Law of One" out of nowhere in my journal every day. After several weeks of writing this out of the blue, I decided to do some research. I found that this law has been written about and channeled through many spiritual masters. The Law of One philosophy is based on the principle that all creation is one and, therefore, inherently connected. Many of my clients who have experienced plant medicine share that they experienced a feeling of being one with everything and everyone, and that this began their spiritual awakening. Many more clients have awakened through their life stories and lessons, without the aid of hallucinogens. For me, it was only necessary to *imagine* that everything is connected to one original thought or mind. If *one original thought* had enough power to create the Universal Field and every reality in it, and we are connected to it, how important might our own thoughts be?

Integrating the Law of One into my everyday reality has left me humble and exhilarated and mirrored my own awakening experience. I am excited about the vastness of our universe and my role in it. This was not always the case.

When I was young, I had a pattern of facing life through my limited lens of survival. I faced my obstacles with fear and stress response. As I have become more self-reflective, I have learned to look at obstacles in a new way. I am more aware of the connections between my challenges and the "non-integrated" aspects of my Creator Matrix. As I have healed these different areas of my Matrix, I have learned to control my thoughts around my challenging storylines and my reactions to them. Now, when a challenge presents itself, I ask, "What thoughts would help me to overcome this?" I can then feel grateful for the lessons and the self-growth they bring me. My challenges have become my greatest teachers. They act as catalysts that force me to go outside of my comfort zone.

As mentioned earlier when I was suffering from postpartum depression, I learned a lot about how to improve my self-care. Once I learned to meditate, I was able to clear my mind daily, which enabled me to take in, retain, and contain new information. Trusting and knowing that everything that happens in my life is for my benefit and for the expansion of my consciousness has helped me to grow and transform. One consequence of clearing and emptying my Creator Matrix was that I became ready for the next step: expanding my capacity as a Creator.

A good friend of mine compares expanding consciousness to "expanding one's container." She taught me that if our container is full, we cannot add anything new. In order to grow your container, you need to have space inside it to do so. This requires you to acknowledge a need to care for your container. For me, the consequence of allowing my consciousness to expand is that my life's focus has become busier with the mystical and magical journey and less busy with the outcome of "getting somewhere" or accumulating material things. I have become much more detached from outcomes. Even though I love the practice of manifesting, enjoying the journey and treasuring the present moment has become far more important to me.

One of my teachers who has helped me master this ability to go inward, get empty, and learn to just "be" has been my youngest daughter, Emma. She was my opposite. At first, I was uncomfortable with her energy because I didn't know how to simply "be." As I observed her quiet, calm, loving nature, I began to connect to a more feminine part of myself. Over time, through her powerful example, I came to understand that when I regularly empty my Creator Matrix and connect to my "beingness," I open up to greater expansion and to divine guidance. I then can ask my higher self anything and know that I will receive immediate guidance that will bring me to my greatest destiny.

This Evolutionary Time

According to some geoscientists, the 1960s began a significant period in history that may be influencing our evolution and our accelerated growth in consciousness (our awakening) as a collective. Some refer to this as the onset of the "Age of Aquarius," which marks the end of the Piscean Age which began around the time of Jesus. Many spiritual thought leaders believe that the Age of Aquarius is the time when the "veil" between our physical world and other dimensions is thinning. This gives us access to a whole new world and a new way of perceiving.

The Piscean Age was dominated by hierarchical structures of top-down leadership and power domination. The Aquarian Age is to be organized by expansional horizontal networks and cooperative leadership. It is the Information Age. Nothing will remain secret, and therefore no one will hold power over others anymore. Since the cultural revolutions of the 1960s, we have been preparing the way through personal transformation, self-reflection, and self-development, as well as major technological advancements in our ability to communicate—most notably, the development of computers and the internet.

Earth "wobbles" on its axis as it orbits the sun. According to NASA, it takes approximately 26,000 years for Earth to complete one full cyclic rotation. This process is known as the "precession of the equinoxes." [1] According to NASA, "Because of the precession wobble of the poles over 26,000 years, all the stars, and other celestial objects, appear to shift west to east at the rate of .014 degree each year (360 degrees in 26,000 years)." [2] As it progresses through the galaxy, Earth will pass through each of the twelve constellations, and the qualities of each constellation will influence both Earth and its inhabitants.

As the Earth orients itself to the galaxy at different "angles," we experience different degrees of light. This affects our bio-individual electromagnetic fields. As previously stated, light is information; therefore, the more light contained in any given space, the more connection and information it is possible to transmit and receive. Some researchers assert that we have just left a period of between 11,000 and 14,000 years of (relative) darkness. With less light comes less information. However, we are now entering a high-frequency galactic photon belt that will last approximately 2,000 years—hence, the association of the Age of Aquarius with enlightenment, information, and increased consciousness.

Research has made it clear that we are influenced by solar flares and Coronal Mass Ejections (CMEs) from the sun. Solar flares are explosions of energy caused by the reorganization of magnetic field lines near sunspots. CMEs are the most powerful solar flares that bring radiation and particles to the Earth's surface. [3] The increase in light from the galactic photon belt and solar flares have a tremendous effect on us at all levels. When CMEs are very strong, they can interfere with the Earth's power grids, causing power outages; similarly, they can disrupt our personal electromagnetic fields. [4] Scientists are still trying to understand the full range of their effects; however, one study found an association between geomagnetic disturbances and an increase in hospital admissions. They also found an increase in existing disease symptoms ranging from mental disorders/suicide, cardiac arrhythmias, heart attacks, increased high blood pressure, and epileptic seizures during periods of solar flares.[5]

These influences also directly impact our current expansion of consciousness due to something called the Schumann Resonance, which is an electromagnetic field around Earth. Many sources during the past several years have even noted that the Schumann Resonance, referred to as the "heartbeat of Mother Earth," for example, has been increasing in frequency from 7.83 Hz to somewhere between 8.5 Hz and 16 Hz. This suggests that both Earth's frequency as well as our own frequencies are increasing. With increased light, more information becomes available to us.

Humans' individual electromagnetic fields range between 5–10 Hz. The Schumann Resonance not only influences telecommunications, but also our brainwaves and many other areas of our human systems, including circadian rhythms, melatonin production, blood pressure, and even reproduction.[6][7] As the Earth's "heartbeat" changes and evolves in response to galactic energies, so too will our own.

Coupled with the increase in light from the galactic photon belt, the changes in the Schumann Resonance and the uptick in solar flares and CMEs are having a tremendous effect on us as individuals. Light is information, and information is light. With more information available to us, our ways of thinking and feeling will shift, perhaps dramatically. Ultimately, these changes will expand our consciousness and allow us to live in and create from a higher level of synergy with the quantum field. When we increase our consciousness, we transition from beta waves to activating our gamma waves in our brain. According to Dr. Joe Dispenza, "Gamma brain waves, which can be more than twice as high as high beta brain waves, represent an aroused state in the brain, however, they are not connected to the survival states of emergency mode, but correlated with a kind of super consciousness and awareness, as well as higher amounts of love and compassion."[8] We will further explore the potential for this new multidimensional reality in Chapter Eleven.

Human Brain Waves

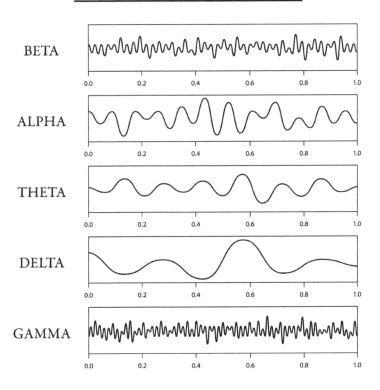

Quantum Science

Consciousness is moving, changing, adapting, transcending, and evolving all the time. As we grow in consciousness, we see more and more of Creation—what we have created individually as well as collectively, as well as what has been and is being created by Universal Source. To be conscious means to be connected to the ever-expanding universe and everything in it.

In order to understand consciousness from a scientific perspective, we need to examine the concepts of perception and observation. We perceive and interpret experiences and our environment through all of our senses. Our five basic senses—sight, hearing, smell, taste, and touch—allow us to connect with the world around us. We can then observe our surroundings and interact with them appropriately. Our perceptions and observations link directly to thoughts and feelings. Sometimes these perceptions and observations can trigger thoughts and emotions connected to visions, biases, memories, genetic information stored in the DNA, and past life stories or memories. Perceptions and observations can be either conscious or unconscious. As we are able to live more in the "now" moment, we begin to make them more conscious. A person's unconscious perception is often driven by a limited "container" that can only manage to contain a smaller amount of information. As we grow in consciousness, our containers become bigger and can contain more information; this empowers us to make different choices.

Our emotions are extremely important in this process of perception and observation because they are stored in our memory and connected to particular experiences. Emotions function like a compass to help us navigate our way through life. They tell us how we are doing. They help us digest, learn, and integrate our life lessons. They also keep us safe by endeavoring to protect us from repeating past or future stories that may cause us harm.

Quantum science has proven that our perception can change the very nature of reality. For example, in the famous Double-Slit Experiment, researchers documented that the behavior of particles changed depending on whether or not they were being observed.[9] This experiment showed that "the observer is an active participant in the fundamental behavior of particles." If our mere *attention* can change the nature of reality, what might our thoughts and intentions do? The researchers were left with an important question that still baffles quantum scientists to this day: "Does the world we take for granted even exist until we perceive it?"

As they search for answers to these questions, quantum scientists are exploring the energy that is at the core of all creation: the quantum field. This has been described as a sort of energetic "soup"—a type of plasma that waits for our instructions to mold and shape itself on a physical level. This plasma is made of strings and strands of light particles that have an innate intelligence within.

As human beings, we can see only some of the connections being made in this field. However, the quantum field sees all connections and possibilities, including those of higher realms of consciousness. This is why many equate the quantum field to Universal Source and pure consciousness.

As mentioned above, we as humans are now expanding our consciousness and increasing our frequencies both personally and collectively. This quantum jump is changing the way we see our reality. At some point in this change, we will be transitioning to higher densities (specifically, from third density to fifth density; this will be further explored in Chapter Eleven).

We all have the capacity to connect to the quantum field. Our bodies, when functioning in an optimal state, are built for it. Part of our evolutionary path on Earth is to relearn how to connect to our higher self and the quantum field, as well as to ground the frequency from these higher realms into our physical matter and reality. When we learn to do this, our awareness will expand. We will see more of our individual reality and connect to more "information"—aka, light particles from the quantum field. Remember, light contains information, therefore light is information.

Akashic Records

Many spiritual masters and leaders throughout history believed that our DNA exists not only on the physical plane but also on the mental plane and in other dimensions. Proving that DNA exists on the physical level was an important task. However, as we are evolving quickly, I am convinced this challenge of proving DNA in other dimensions will be humanity's next frontier.

Tibetan monks refer to this "invisible" DNA as *Akash*, meaning "astral light," and is each soul's record of karma. However, it now seems to be much more: a field of recorded personalized information and data that contains our deepest inner wisdom as well as the secrets of our past and future selves. The Akash is a sort of "etheric living library" that connects with your physical DNA on the earthly plane.[10] The DNA as a whole seems to function multidimensionally on the physical, mental, and etheric/spiritual level, but the Akash exists on a mental or etheric plane. This etheric level can be looked at as an electromagnetic field of energy or a library of light. When we connect to this wisdom, it can guide us through our earthly experiences. In theosophy and the school of anthroposophy, it is believed that Akashic Records are encoded vibrationally into space, like a hologram of data.

Everything we have ever said, done, and experienced in the past, present, and future has been recorded in the Akash. This includes all thoughts, words, deeds, and memories. Looking at DNA as a multidimensional record gives us a new understanding of DNA and our connection to it. We are influenced by our past, present, and future selves through this library of information. This includes all positive and/or negative genetic tendencies as well as any unresolved issues or imbalances that may have been passed on through generations.

The Akash holds a space for each soul as a sovereign and unique Creator—like a universal passport of storylines and experiences. Our life lessons are made unique by our past genetics (Akashic Records), fears, experiences, emotional intelligence, and personality. Each soul creates their own storylines, and each is connected to the collective energy of all.

Many of us, as we are awakening, are doing the spiritual work of offloading negative unresolved karma, and coming to understand we are constantly influencing, impacting, and changing the multidimensional field. As a result, we are feeling and experiencing a "lightening" of our entire being and simultaneously claiming our tremendous power to change our life path and influence our life stories.

Creating Safety

As we work on offloading and unblocking, we become aware of which stories leave us feeling unsafe. Our life lessons on Earth can often shake up our feelings of safety on all levels of our Creator Matrix. We can be challenged through our stories to feel safe physically if our health is less than optimal, or if we are in a physically abusive relationship, going through a divorce, have an accident, fight in or live through a war, and many other storylines. We can be challenged to feel safe mentally if we are connected to darker experiences and our system is overloaded. Finally, we can be challenged to feel safe spiritually if we are confused about why we are here on Earth and what life and living truly mean.

Many of these challenges can cause us to struggle and function in pure survival mode. This was my reality as a child. As I've shared, my childhood was rather chaotic, and the energies on the planet had me feeling very unsafe. My sister, Christin, helped me through this period of my life. We shared a bedroom, and her presence of unconditional love anchored me. From her, I learned the valuable lesson that no person in our lives is there by accident or coincidence. Each of the Creators we co-create with is essential for our development. As Maslow's Hierarchy of Needs tells us, we cannot expand our reality (consciousness), step into our true power, or attain self-actualization if we feel unsafe.

We are able to create safety by learning to feel safe within ourselves in all situations, regardless of our past storylines. This is why it is important to heal those past aspects of ourselves that felt "unsafe," digest any lingering emotions, and expand into new storylines.

Consciousness, Light, and Manifesting

Learning that light and consciousness are interconnected was exciting for me. This information led me to another question: "What is the relationship between consciousness, light, and manifesting?"

Our awareness and consciousness determine what we focus on and where we direct our energy. What we focus on expands; in this way, consciousness influences how we impact our energetic field. We can therefore say that consciousness eventually moves energy into a form that we manifest. As we increase our consciousness, we are also increasing our frequency to a higher level which contains more light and information. As we learn to maintain this higher frequency, we will naturally bring into form situations and experiences that mirror that frequency. We can choose our experiences and influence our creations by mirroring the frequency we wish to experience. If we mirror the lower emotional frequencies and thought forms of lack, we will attract more of this. However, if we mirror the higher emotional frequencies connected to thought forms of abundance and love, we will attract more of these as well. If we mirror higher frequencies of loving relationships, this will influence who turns up in our lives.

The highest frequencies and emotions we can experience for the life that we seek on Planet Earth are love, joy, trust, authenticity, and peace. As we attune to these emotions and their related thought forms, we become integrated with them and attract new experiences. It is not enough to simply think a new thought and manifest; one must consciously focus on that thought and feel the experience of having it in order for it to manifest. Thinking it, knowing it, *and* feeling it are essential to this process.

Underpinning it all is our ability to contain what we wish to manifest. We will not manifest what we cannot contain. If we want to manifest a job with a higher salary and go to the interview with the dominant frequency of unworthiness or fear that we will not be able to do the job well, we will not get the job. If we live our life in fear, we live a life of avoidance. When we are overwhelmed with the responsibility of attracting the thing we wish to manifest, we will often sabotage ourselves. Ultimately, a lack of self-worth and self-love are the catalysts behind this. How effective can we be as Creators if we feel unworthy and are not able to love ourselves? Would you consciously follow such a Creator?

When we work through our fears, our consciousness will suddenly shift to allow new possibilities. These possibilities, if held consistently, become a "new version of ourselves" that we can align with. Knowing how amazing we truly are as humans and realizing how worthy we really are is the most significant step in raising our consciousness. As we learn to do this, we become inspired to trust and love ourselves completely. We learn to expect "miracles" and change the possibilities we will experience.

In the coming chapters we will explore this further—but for now, let's look at what neuroscience has to say about consciousness.

Neuroscience and Consciousness

Neuroscientists have been trying for decades to understand where consciousness comes from. During the 1970s and 1980s, many scientists were focused on the cognitive sciences and were reluctant to look at consciousness itself, believing it to be linked to subjective perception rather than quantum expression. Moreover, anything that looked beyond the physical and mechanical operations of the brain was considered a "soft science" and not evidence-based.

By the 1990s, further technological advancements improved researchers' brain scanning abilities with MRIs and EEGs, and many scientists began to explore where, when, and how the brain processes information. Today, neuroscientists have clearly shown that thoughts are transmitted through neural networks in the brain, but there is still some debate as to which neural networks and areas of the brain are involved in consciousness itself. In fact, research is showing that consciousness is not limited to one area of the brain.

In her 2019 article, "Decoding the Nature of Consciousness," Emily Sohn wrote, "It has become increasingly clear, however, that consciousness is not confined to only one region of the brain. Various cells and pathways are engaged, depending on what is being perceived or the type of perception that is involved."[11]

Some brave researchers are questioning the essence of consciousness itself, and wondering if it resides in our physical matter at all. New theories point to the idea that each human being has their own electromagnetic field that is superimposed upon and connected to their physical body. This suggests that the brain's electromagnetic field can influence the conscious integration of information via the neural networks. Moreover, it supposes that consciousness is a manifestation of the brain's electromagnetic field, and that this field is capable of integrating vast quantities of information into a single physical system, thereby accounting for the binding of consciousness.[12]

However, the most important outcome of this research is the knowledge that our subjective observations and foci impact what information we send, receive, integrate, and ultimately experience. This, again, brings the power of consciousness back to us as Creators. What we focus on expands. How we choose to write our story, which beliefs we choose to nurture, what emotions we choose to feel, and what words we allow ourselves to express will influence what and how we create.

Using our Intuition

As we mentioned above, our five senses help us perceive our reality. However, these senses exist on a physical level. Many other senses exist on the levels of mind and spirit.

You've likely heard the term "the sixth sense." Some also refer to this as a "gut feeling" or a "knowing." I call it *intuition*. This "knowingness" can come from an accumulation of our past learned experiences, information from a larger field of knowledge (the Universal Field), emotional and motor neurons (empathy), or from our soul's knowledge (heart center). Sometimes we just need to get our brain out of the way. We can get our greatest "a-ha" moments as we are doing something like meditation or running that distracts us and allows our brain to take a break and wander.

Our intuition develops as our consciousness grows, and as we learn to trust and interpret signals from our environment with accuracy. As we gain this ability, we become aware of how our personal biases can change our interpretation and learn to keep our biases in check.

Remember also that our amygdala is constantly checking—through our five senses—whether we are safe or unsafe in any given situation. As we develop our intuition, we can learn to recognize whether we have been triggered to feel unsafe, or whether we truly are unsafe. If we have been triggered, we can learn to control our reaction.

The most important factor is to practice using your skill of "knowingness" and to learn to trust it. In my experience, the more we trust this ability, the more information we will gain access to. Intuition is deeply connected to the electromagnetic field of the heart, and our ability to "feel" what our five senses cannot perceive. In essence, our sixth sense is our ability to perceive and glean information from *energy*.

Over the years, I've learned to follow and trust my intuition. When I try to explain that I simply have a "knowing" about something, many logical, left-brain dominant people find it difficult to understand that I could know something without knowing how I know. However, the definition of "intuition" is "the ability to understand something instinctively, without the need for conscious reasoning." So actually, it's quite logical that intuitive guidance should be received as "knowingness," because there is literally no other way for intuition to operate.

I connect to my intuition as an "inner voice" that guides me, and I usually feel it in my solar plexus. I use my intuition when making any kind of important decision. I think of the problem and the potential options available to me, and then focus on my feelings to guide me in making the best decision for myself. Most of the time, this "inner voice" guides me through feeling: the choice that feels "lighter" is usually the right one, and often will present notably fewer obstacles. For example, when I was living in the United States with my husband Frans, he received two job offers. One was at an office in the World Trade Center in New York City, and the other required him to move to the Netherlands in order to work in the family business. Frans said that he didn't care which he accepted, and that it was up to me. It would have been much easier for me to encourage him to choose New York. My entire family and most of my friends lived on the East Coast. There were further work opportunities for me there as well, and I had always wanted to work in New York City. However, when I looked inward and felt the two possibilities, New York felt very heavy, while the Netherlands felt light. It did not take me long to recognize that we needed to move to Europe. I actually had to go against what I thought I wanted and instead choose what I felt and knew was the best decision for our future.

Not too long after our move, the 9/11 attacks decimated the World Trade Center. I needed no further proof that I should trust my "knowingness." This ability to transcend the limited knowing of our five senses is the beginning of multidimensional living.

I have also used my intuition to perceive danger and to protect myself and my family. One time, in the middle of the day, a man entered my house as my two children were sleeping upstairs. As I greeted him on the staircase, knowing full well that his intentions were not good, I smiled and said, "How are you? Maybe you're lost? May I show you the door so you can find your way?" As I remained calm, he returned my smile and walked out the door with me. I said goodbye and subsequently called the police. It turned out he was a major drug dealer in the area that the police had been searching for. My inner voice guided me to remain calm and act without fear. This derailed his malicious intentions.

It's my belief that, when we listen to our inner knowing, we are being guided by a power beyond what we understand. We can all develop this ability—and many people utilize this ability unconsciously as part of their daily lives. In an article published on their website, titled, "Intuition—It's More Than a Feeling," the Association for Psychological Science (APS) asserts,

"From Albert Einstein to Oprah Winfrey, many top leaders ascribe their success to having followed their intuition. New research shows how going with our gut instincts can help guide us to faster, more accurate decisions. Intuition — the idea that individuals can make successful decisions without deliberate analytical thought — has intrigued philosophers and scientists since at least the times of the ancient Greeks."[13]

134

In fact, new research shows that our "gut instinct" is correct an average of 80 percent of the time.[14] Another study published in the journal *Psychological Science,* entitled "Measuring Intuition: Nonconscious Emotional Information Boosts Decision Accuracy and Confidence," further supports this. [15] Other organizations, such as the HeartMath Institute, have studied the connection between intuition and our heart; HeartMath has developed knowledge and tools that support an intuitive connection with the heart.[16]

As we grow in consciousness, many more of us are recognizing how to use our intuition—and it's a good thing, because our modern systems demand that we receive, analyze, and act on more complex and innovative information than is available through our five senses.

At this time, we know of seven senses related to advanced intuition skills that each human will mature into. These intuitive senses involve developing our telepathic skills, which means that we are learning new ways to perceive and connect to our environment outside of our five physical senses. During my spiritual awakening, I noticed a quickening of these psychic abilities; this has also happened for many of my clients. For some people, this process can be rather shocking as they suddenly become incredibly aware of other people's dramas, feelings, untruths, and life stories. When this happened to me, I was excited at first, but quickly became exhausted and overwhelmed by the sheer degree of information I was receiving. It was an information overload, and I felt as though I was invading others' privacy. I now only connect to someone's "field" of information when they ask for it and have come to me for a healing or coaching session.

The seven "new" senses that accompany an expansion of consciousness are: clairvoyance, claircognition, clairaudience, clairsentience, claircognizance, clairalience, and clairgustance. Many people on the planet have been developing these abilities, and others (new children or light workers) have come to Earth with them fully developed.

Clair Cognition refers to the ability to learn to follow your gut feeling or psychic knowing. This is a gift that many have and are developing at this time. It is the "knowingness" I described above.

Clairvoyance literally means "one who sees clearly," and refers to the ability to see without our eyes.

Clairaudience, "clear hearing," is the ability to hear without using our ears and receive intuitive guidance through hearing; in other words, to hear what is not being said, to listen between the lines, and to hear our own inner voice. Some people even hear voices and sounds from beyond the physical realm if they have developed this ability, such as the voices of angels or other divine entities.

Clairsentience is to feel things beyond touch. This is the capacity to have heightened sensitivity through our tactile abilities—to feel frequencies of energy, to feel the density of energy, and to feel what others feel in and through our bodies. An example of this may be physical sensations like chills that let us know we are on the right path with our thoughts and feelings about something. In fact, this skill developed quickly as I began helping myself and others heal energetically.

Claircognizance is the ability to transcend time and space. This is about knowing things in the future and past timelines.

Clairalience means "heightened smell" and refers to someone who is able to smell scents of things that are not physically there in the vicinity with them.

Clairgustance refers to "clear tasting" and means a person can taste something like herbs or foods when that person isn't even eating. Many psychics and medical intuitives have developed this ability.

It's possible that you have already had experiences of these seven "etheric" senses in your life. If not, you can still cultivate them through the process of expanding your consciousness and paying attention to the feelings and sensations in your body, mind, and energy fields, especially during those times when you are called to make decisions. Once you begin to receive information directly from the quantum field, your capacity and possibilities will expand enormously.

Your Conscious Expansion

As we grow in consciousness, we learn to be the observer. As the observer, we may choose how we will react to any given situation, remembering that our thought forms and emotions impact our environment. Love in our storylines will bring more love to us, just as hate will bring more hate to us. We always have a choice where we want to hang out. Our consciousness affects how we direct our energy and what we will attract and bring into physical reality.

Manifesting is the process by which we summon and integrate with the field to bring an intention into form. With more information becoming available to us, our way of thinking and feeling will be shifting, and ultimately expanding our consciousness. We are becoming aware that our very thoughts are the building blocks of reality. Thoughts are like seeds that influence what future timelines we will manifest. At this time on Earth, we are changing our reality, which means that the old systems around us (our environment and societal systems) will naturally change and adjust to our new expanded thoughts and new frequencies. Our changed consciousness will attract new systems that align with our new paradigm.

So, how can you become more conscious today and align your thoughts and emotions to what you wish to experience?

In the next chapter, we will further explore more about energy and the science behind this phenomenon.

Chapter Summary

- The base of consciousness is energy. It is life force, the force that allows all creation to exist.

- We are spiritual beings having a physical experience.

- Consciousness is the state of knowing oneself or "knowingness" in general.

- We live in an evolutionary time, the Age of Aquarius, a time of enlightenment, information, and increased consciousness, with the Earth entering a high-frequency photon belt in this part of Earth's orbit around the sun.

- Light is information and information is light. With the increased light from the photon belt , more information follows, which will shift our ways of thinking and feeling, which will ultimately expand our consciousness and allow us to live in and create from a higher level of synergy with the quantum field.

- Quantum science has proven that our perception can change the very nature of reality.

- The quantum field is the energy at the core of all creation. It is a type of plasma, made of strings and strands of light particles that have an innate intelligence.

- The quantum field waits for our instructions to mold and shape itself on a physical level.

- The quantum jump in frequency, both personally and collectively, is changing the way we will see our reality, transitioning to higher densities.

- Part of our evolutionary path on Earth is to relearn how to connect to our higher self and the quantum field, as well as ground the frequency from these higher realms into our physical matter and reality.

- We cannot expand our reality (consciousness) and step into our true power as well as develop our self-actualization and awareness if we feel unsafe. We are able to create safety by feeling safe in all situations.

- Awareness and consciousness determine what we focus on and where we direct our energy. What we focus on expands. Consciousness moves energy into a form that we manifest.

- What we bring into form and manifest mirrors our frequency. We can choose our experiences and influence our creations by mirroring the frequency we wish to experience. Manifesting requires thinking and consciously focusing on that thought, feeling the experience of having it already and being able to contain what we wish to manifest.

- With a lack of self-worth and self-love we can self-sabotage our manifestations.

- As we learn to trust and love ourselves completely, we learn to expect miracles and change the possibilities we will experience.

- Our subjective observations and foci impact what information we send, receive, integrate, and ultimately experience. What we focus on expands. How we choose to write our story, which beliefs we choose to nurture, what emotions we choose to feel, and the words we allow ourselves to express will influence what and how we create.

- Intuition is deeply connected to the electromagnetic field of the heart and our ability to "feel" or sense what our five senses cannot perceive. Our sixth sense is our ability to perceive and glean information from energy.

- As we are growing in consciousness, we are waking up and recognizing how to use our intuition. We will develop our advanced intuitive senses, including telepathic skills and other senses, like clairvoyance. clairaudience, clairsentience, claircognizance, clairalience, and clairgustance.

Chapter Six

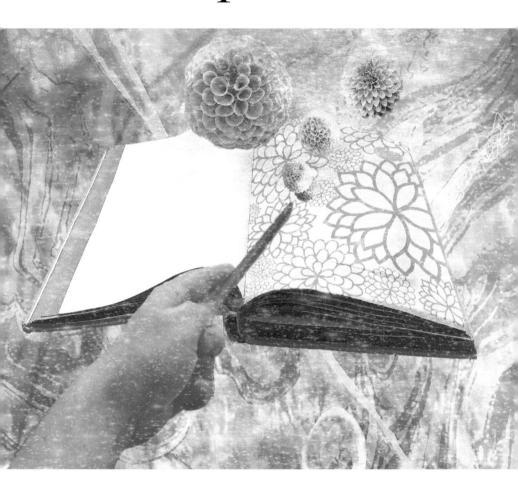

How are you directing your energy?
How are you using your magic wand?

"Matter is Energy ... Energy is Light ...
We are all Light Beings."

- Albert Einstein

CHAPTER SIX

Energy

As a young girl, I was highly sensitive and highly reactive, both physically and emotionally. I did not know what was fueling my extreme sensitivity—only that I was easily frightened and overwhelmed and was not fully understood by others in my environment. My ideas were often difficult for others to connect with and for this reason, I had difficulty connecting. It was a little later in my life that I began to meet other like-minded people who shared many similar ideas, and I felt more at home.

I was born in the 1960s and, in addition to all the political and racial unrest happening at the time, we were also subjected to daily chatter about the Vietnam War. As I shared in the Introduction, my parents were activists, and at the same time my dad moved from job to job searching for one he felt a passion for. We moved from South Bend, Indiana, to Midland Michigan, to Fort Wayne, Indiana, to Saginaw, Michigan, to Washington D.C.—and, during all those moves, my parents managed to have six children in seven years. As you can imagine, their marriage was under stress. This created turbulence for me as I could not ground myself, find my place, or feel my worth. Luckily, my siblings became my best friends, and this helped me to feel connected and accepted.

As the eldest child, I naturally took on a lot of responsibility, and I had an empathic ability that was extreme. I was able to see and feel what others felt. Being unaware of this at the time, I unconsciously took on the emotions, pain, and suffering of others. The emotional "baggage" I was carrying for others began to create physical pain within my own body. I dealt with routine stomach pains and constant sore throats. I also began to feel misplaced fear and anxiety that I was unable to control. Unfortunately, my parents were far too busy to handle this as they had many issues of their own. Without my bond with my siblings, this would have been unbearable.

As I grew into adulthood, the anxiety became so great that I needed to seek professional help. As a nurse, I was always terrified of hurting someone (which was highly inconvenient at work). I was also incredibly aware of others' physical, emotional, and mental pain. Their stories seemed to follow me around—from the friends who had cancer, to the teacher who committed suicide, to my patients in the hospital. On my first nursing ward, my superior picked up on my fear of harming others and, in an effort to make me more "practical," exacerbated my insecurities.

I was unable to pinpoint where this fear of doing harm was coming from. However, after working with a kinesiologist, José, and an Ayurvedic psychiatrist, Dr. Levin, I began to learn about energy—and, in particular, about how the body stores, moves, and incorporates energy on all levels.

This learning was compounded when I had my third child. After her birth, I noticed that my physical body from three births and all the years in nursing was depleted. I was looking for new solutions to improve my physical health, and for all my clients the lesson is that finding health and wellness is never about one thing. A Creator Matrix on all levels must be nourished. I had already been experimenting with many forms of complementary medicine during those years, like acupuncture, cranial-osteopathy, classic homeopathy, Ayurvedic medicine, and meditation. I noticed a gradual increase in energy and well-being with all of them. I learned a lot during this period about nutrition and I will further discuss this in Chapters Eight and Nine. One modality in particular impacted my understanding of the importance of our energetic system: Reconnective Healing' and the work of Dr. Eric Pearl.

It started when my sister-in-law, Eveline, called to inform me that she had bought me an experiential birthday gift; namely, a three-week course learning to heal with my hands. I remember rolling my eyes and saying, "I have no interest in learning to heal with my hands." I wasn't interested in learning to be an energy healer at the time; my nursing background still led me to harbor a fair amount of skepticism around things I couldn't see or touch. I had not yet made the connection between our energetic systems and our health and wellness. However, she convinced me to join her and give it a try.

To my surprise, just being in the presence of this teacher created a shift in me. I could feel frequencies circulating through my hands and in my entire biological system. After the first class, I was amazed at how much lighter and happier I felt. I also started to help others with these techniques, and many people experienced the same reactions I had. I went on to study more with Dr. Pearl and became a practitioner of Reconnective Healing.

Ironically, my sister-in-law did not feel these frequencies. We laugh about it to this day as she has often connected me to spiritual pathways. I now understand that we all have different gifts, and it will become increasingly important for us to share these with one another for the benefit of mankind as we evolve.

What is Energy?

In the last few chapters, we've learned about how our stories, beliefs, thought forms, and consciousness influence our reality and impact our ability to act as a Creator in our lives.

Now, we're going to look more deeply at the mechanics behind all of these things—quantum mechanics, to be specific. And we will begin by exploring *energy*.

As Dr. Pearl writes on his website, "An optimal state of balance

... results from interacting with a fully comprehensive spectrum of frequencies consisting of Energy, Light and Information."[1] Energy connects all parts of us. It is present at all levels of our being—body, mind, and spirit—and is essential to our experience of consciousness and well-being. In fact, it is impossible to experience the fullness of our power as Creators without having an understanding of how to work with and optimize our energy.

So, what *is* energy, and how does it impact our ability to achieve optimal well-being and be the Creator in our lives?

Many of us use the term "energy" loosely. We think of it as something we have or don't have, depending on the circumstance. We say things like, "I have no energy," "He has the best energy," or, "Her energy is all over the place today." But how many of us truly know and understand that we *are* energy—and that the actions of our thoughts, feelings, and physical body serve to direct that energy?

We humans, at our core, are energy having a temporary stay in a human body, as I've mentioned before. We can illustrate this concept using the analogy of getting into a car. The car is the physical container that holds the spiritual field that can drive it around. Our bodies are likewise containers for our energy.

Einstein's Law of Conservation of Energy tells us a little bit about energy: that it can be neither created nor destroyed, only changed from one form to another. Merriam-Webster's definition of energy offers further clarity, stating that energy is "a fundamental entity of nature that is transferred between parts of a system in the production of physical change within the system."

Common forms of energy include heat, sound, light, gravity, and kinetic (motion) energy. As humans, we are a combination of energy stored as mass in physical form, energy in motion (such as our body heat, the electric synapses of our brains, and the sound we can produce), and energy as potential. We are a noun and a verb; we are yang and yin.

What is Quantum Mechanics?

Let us take a brief look at the relationship between energy and matter. In order to do this, we need to take a closer look at quantum mechanics. The science of quantum mechanics explains how the universe works on a sub-atomic level. The term "quantum mechanics" is often used interchangeably with "quantum physics" or "quantum theory." However, "mechanics" refers to the part of physics that explains how things move—in particular, how subatomic particles move.[2] Much of quantum mechanics is focused on the behaviors of matter and light on the subatomic scale.[3] Ultimately, this new quantum world is looking at how we, as Creators, can influence our reality. It further examines how our thought forms can and will affect the subatomic world and beyond.

When I began to research this on the subatomic level, I was struck by the idea that this level consists predominantly of "empty" space. Seen from the subatomic level, our bodies are 99.9999999% empty space interspersed with tiny bits of matter.[4] All of that space and matter are contained within an energetic field. Quantum mechanics strives to understand how matter influences this field of space and how this space, in turn, influences matter. As we learned in Chapter Five, a person's perceptions and observations will influence what the quantum field will manifest. Alongside empty space, energy is transmitted through sound and light. Light and sound are both made of waves and are transported through vibrations. Light is manifested as photons at the physical level.

In our body, mind, and spirit matrix, the material and non-material worlds interact in a complex interplay. This is much like a dance as we co-create with the field of all possibilities. We are energy and we are all connected. As consciousness is evolving, it is becoming increasingly apparent to us that we are energy, and therefore connected to everything and everyone, including worlds and dimensions we cannot see with our human eyes. If you think about it, there are many things we cannot see with our eyes. This principle is echoed in the Electric Universe Theory, which posits that electricity is the driving force that connects all things.[5] Atoms hold electromagnetic waves of light and information. Everything in the universe is made up of these electromagnetic fields of energy and has its own frequency.

According to an increasing body of scientific evidence, the non-material elements of our human existence are composed of energy. Thought forms are energy, as are emotions, beliefs, and attitudes. Taken together, our material bodily processes and our energy system make up a human energy field. Scientists are now proving the existence of this human energy field and its relationship to health and wellness. They describe it as a biofield that is both electromagnetic and biophotonic in nature. A 2015 study published in *Global Advances in Health and Medicine* defines the term *biofield* as "a field of energy and information ... that regulates the homeodynamic function of living organisms." The study further states that, "The evidence for the existence of the biofield holds the promise of significant growth in scientific understanding and for developing applications in medicine, health, and healing."[6]

The existence of the human biofield is further explored through what researchers have dubbed the "phantom leaf effect." Through Kirlian photography, the energy or "aura" of various leaves were rendered clearly visible. This experiment went on to show that the biofield of the leaf remained even after part of the leaf was severed from the original whole.[7]

These fields are self-regulating and influence cellular health and the organization of the system as a whole. I am happy that science is now looking at these powerful connections between our energetic system and the healing experiences that I have witnessed in my healing work for decades.

Our human energy field connects to the quantum energy field, as it is the origin of our power source. The quantum field fuels the possibility for connection and is what we term the God force, Source energy, quantum field, Universal Field, and/or Zero Point Field. To put it another way, we must regularly connect to a power source in order to rejuvenate, much like an electrical device needs to connect to a power grid in order to recharge. A device can function for a while on a battery, but eventually it will need to be recharged in order to function optimally.

In Isaac Newton's world, everything seemed measurable and predictable. As scientists study the quantum, however, they are learning that much of it is not measurable or predictable. The field has been compared to a "bubbling soup of possibilities." This is what we plug into when we access the quantum field.

One of the main principles of quantum physics is the Heisenberg Uncertainty Principle. This principle questions how the quantum field behaves and how it can be measured. All matter has a rest energy at its base before it is activated by our thought forms. As our thought forms connect to the quantum field, they begin to influence what will be manifested from that field in different forms of matter. Matter can be interchanged between forms of solid, liquid, and gas. According to Dr. Joe Dispenza, scientists are discovering a fourth state known as "plasma," which is the state of possibility before matter is manifested. He states, "Plasma makes up as much as 99 percent of all matter. You can think of plasma as the connective tissue of the unseen world."[8] In other words, before the planets became matter, they were plasma. Before a human embryo is conceived, it is plasma. Plasma can be perceived through electromagnetic fields.

Thought forms are referred to as "scalar waves". They travel faster than the speed of light and transcend space and time as we know it. These thought forms have different electromagnetic frequencies which create fields of information. Information is connected throughout the universe on all levels of mind, body, and spirit, and impacts the design of the structures and the information sent. Plasma is the substance that is formed into geometric structures in a process right before matter comes into form. According to Dr. Dispenza, "As these waves of energy slow down to become matter, at a certain point, just before they turn into solid three-dimensional structures, plasma is organized into complex geometric patterns that serve as the blueprints of matter."[9]

Sacred geometry looks at the blueprint of matter, it looks at how the fundamental structures are organized. The universe is intelligent and has self-organizing mechanisms that act as a template for all creation.

These templates are geometrically, beautifully, coherently organized and expressed by Prime Creator and co-Creators. Many cultures throughout history have studied these patterns and their mathematical equations and codes. Our very DNA has codes and is organized as a living library. We as Creators affect the field by our coherence and clarity. If our Creator Matrix is disordered or chaotic, then our creations will be affected. The geometric patterns will be misaligned and of low frequency.

The work of Masaru Emoto, with which you may be familiar, shows that water is shaped by the environments to which it is exposed, including the thoughts, words, and emotions present in those environments. His work shows that our very thoughts influence water, creating either beautiful, coherent structures of high-frequency light or darker, chaotic structures of low-frequency light. Each of these creations carries an electromagnetic field of information. This made me ask myself, "What kind of impact am I having on the world around me by the thoughts and emotions I generate? Am I contributing to a more coherent and beautiful world, or to a darker, more chaotic world?"

An electromagnetic field has both electric and magnetic properties and surrounds a person, animal, plant, or object with an electrical charge. Its behavior is determined by the wavelengths and frequencies of the energies being generated within the field.[10] According to the HeartMath Institute, "The heart is the most powerful source of electromagnetic energy in the human body, producing the largest rhythmic electromagnetic field of any of the body's organs. The heart's electrical field is about sixty times greater in amplitude than the electrical activity generated by the brain."[11]

Our health seems to be dependent on how our electromagnetic field is vibrating, flowing, and directing the energy at the physical level of our bodies. These fields hold a blueprint for a pattern that influences how matter will be structured. This structure then influences function. The different planes of the human energetic field, as we learned in Chapter One, are physical, emotional, mental, and spiritual. These different planes all affect each other as well as the overall health of the field. Some people refer to our body's electromagnetic field as our aura.

Understanding Albert Einstein's description of energy (that it cannot be created or destroyed, but can only change form), we as humans are learning that we can control, to a greater extent than we have ever realized, how our human form shall exist and change. Through our stories, beliefs, habits, choices, and level of consciousness, our energy field can become altered, blocked, and depleted—or it can be restored, rebalanced, grounded, and reinvigorated.

When our energy field is blocked, we may experience pain on a physical level, sadness and anger on an emotional level, or even a feeling of disconnection from our soul, our essence, or Universal Source on a spiritual level.

One thing is certain: we, as humans on Earth, *are* energy beings. We also happen to be using our physical vehicles (bodies) to have experiences that allow us to connect to, manage, and master our energy fields. The higher the frequency of our vibration, the higher our energy levels and vitality. Moreover, the higher our individual frequencies, the more we will resonate with similar frequencies within the Universal Field. Knowing this is a starting point for taking charge of our own health and happiness.

The Body Meridians and the Seven Chakras

Our energy fields flow through us and maintain our life force and health. In Eastern traditions, this force is called chi, qi, ki, or prana. Our overall energy field is referred to by many as our aura.

Energy as a part of wellness and Creatorship has been understood for thousands of years. Traditional Chinese Medicine describes an energy system within our bodies in which chi (qi) flows through our meridians and chakras. The twelve meridians act as energetic pathways in the body. In addition to our meridians (known as "nadis" or "nadi lines" in Ayurveda) we also know that there are seven energy centers or portals in our human body that connect to Universal Source energy—aka, the Field. The word *chakra* means "wheel of energy" in Sanskrit.

In essence, our chakras are vortices of energy, and represent different expressions of energy in our bodies.

Here is a brief overview of the seven chakras and the energies they govern.

- The root chakra (muladhara) is located at the base of the spine and is represented by the color red. It holds the energy of safety and belonging.

- The sacral chakra (svadhisthana) is located just below the navel and is represented by the color orange. It holds the energies of creativity, sexuality, and emotion.

- The solar plexus chakra (manipura) is located just below the sternum and is represented by the color yellow or gold. It holds the energy of personal power, autonomy, individuality, and the ego.

- The heart chakra (anahata) is located in the center of the chest and is represented by the color green or pink. It holds the energy of love, connection, and unity.

- The throat chakra (vishuddha) is located in the center of the throat and is represented by the color blue. It holds the energy of communication, truth, and manifesting the inner realms into the material world.

- The third eye chakra (ajna) is located just above the brows in the center of the forehead and is represented by the color indigo. It holds the energy of mental clarity, perception, and discernment.

- The crown chakra (sahasrara) is located at the top (crown) of the head and is represented by the color violet or white. It is the place where divine light and information from Universal Source enters our bodies and communicates with our human energy field.

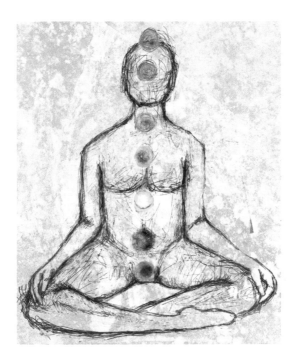

Our material system of genes, cells, organs, and limbs is comple-
mented by an electromagnetic energy system. We must remember that
we are spiritual beings coming into a physical body. Many healers have
spoken about the different "bodies" within the body—namely, the physical body, emotional body, mental body, and the spiritual (soul level) body.
All of these aspects of ourselves come together to make us multidimensional beings. At death, our energetic field separates from our body.

Our chakras impact our human energy field by bringing energy
into our system and circulating it within that system—or, by blocking
energy from entering or circulating within our system. The more the
chakra system is blocked by stress, undigested emotions, or unhelpful
beliefs, the greater the chance of developing an imbalance or disease.
The more "open" we are—meaning, our chakras and meridians are
unblocked and allowing energy to flow freely within our electromagnetic field—the healthier we can become, physically, emotionally, mentally, and spiritually. Just like blood flows freely through our arteries

and veins when we are healthy, so must our energy field flow. If our blood vessels become clogged, we may suffer a blood clot, heart attack, or stroke. If our energetic field gets bogged down by a buildup of undigested emotions or by spiritual stagnation, our meridians and chakras can become blocked in much the same way. This energetic blockage can eventually lead to physical blockages if not managed.

There are many modalities that can assist with opening energy channels and processing energetic blockages in all areas of the body. These include acupuncture, Ayurveda therapy, neurofeedback therapy, family constellation therapy, osteopathy, kinesiology, orthomolecular therapy, classic homeopathy, reflexology, massage, energy healing, reiki, color therapy, Polarity Healing, and aromatherapy, to name a few. All offer ways to create and maintain balance both energetically and physically. Good lifestyle habits, such as practicing yoga and meditation, journaling, breathwork, or exercise can also support energetic balance.

As I grow in consciousness, I have learned to keep my energy field flowing and in high frequency through daily techniques of meditation, chanting, and most recently sound ball exercises. These practices keep my entire Creator Matrix in harmony and balance. With all the change and chaos around us, it is important to replenish and nourish our energy fields. Recently, I attended a consciousness retreat with world-renowned visionaries including Dr. Shamini Jain. Through simple exercises like humming, we learned to shift our field quickly and easily. We experienced that, by making these sounds, we can both clear blockages instantly and uplift our entire system. When we do not feel well, our energetic system (aura) is contracted and small, and when we feel optimally well our field is expanded and joyful.

I also make a habit of regularly connecting to the Universal Field by opening my crown chakra to receive high-frequency light (white light) and grounding myself to Mother Earth. I am convinced that if everyone could do these daily practices, the planet would become much more peaceful and loving. When I open the channels in this way, I also receive information from the Field and Mother Earth, which helps me navigate my day and focus my intentions more directly.

The Law of Vibration

People often talk about the Law of Attraction and understand that they must attract what they really want in their life by aligning their frequency with their desires. Frequency and vibration are the foundation of the Law of Attraction. The Law of Attraction is based on the Principle of Vibration, which states that nothing rests—that everything moves and is always in motion.[12] As mentioned above, our thoughts and feelings directly influence our rate of vibration. Our rate of vibration influences our electromagnetic field, and our field influences what we attract into our reality and how it manifests.

Dr. Randolph Stone, doctor of Osteopathy, Naturopathy, and Chiropractic, also believes in the Principle of Vibration. He writes, "The energy rhythm of Life must be kept moving through every part of it or it suffers, as well as its four polarized varieties of this element, embodied in four states or kinds of matter: Fire (heat, warmth, energy); Air (air, oxygen, gas); Earth (solids, food); Water (liquids and beverage)."

Dr. Stone believes that energy runs through the body, and that this same energy runs through all creation and the universe. At the basic level, energy either attracts or repels, moving out from Source and returning to Source. Source is the ether and is the only unmanifested element. The mind sits between soul and matter. In order to be healthy and well, all of these elements must be free to move and be in balance with one another. Once all is in motion, our thoughts connect to the Universal Field and condense energy, manifesting it into form.

I often use Dr. Stone's polarity techniques to help people heal and rebalance. I have come to appreciate that healing our Creator Matrix is a beautiful dance between the connection and flow of our life force energy (chi/qi/prana) and the four elements that vibrate uniquely, eventually forming into structures of matter. When the energy of the body is able to revitalize and restore, it is in motion and healthy. Dr Stone refers to this as "wireless energy"—the foundation of equalized current flow for health.[13] If there are blockages in the energetic system, there can be an over- or under-stimulation that can change the frequency and the flow; this can lead to imbalance and disease.

FREQUENCIES AND PHYSICAL HEALTH

Our thoughts, our emotions, and our physical bodies play a big role in creating our bio-individual frequency—but when I say, "Everything has a frequency," I mean *everything*. Viruses, animals, bacteria, cells, and even atoms have their own frequencies, and their frequencies interact with ours as we navigate life on Planet Earth. What is frequency actually? Frequency is a measurement of how often a recurring event such as a wave occurs in a measurement of time.

Nicola Tesla is quoted as saying, "If you could eliminate certain outside frequencies that interfered in our bodies, we would have greater resistance toward disease." Dr. Robert O. Becker, author of *The Body Electric*, explains that humans have an electrical frequency and that our health is in direct correlation with that frequency. Bruce Tainio, researcher and founder of Tainio Technology & Technique, Inc., created the BT3 Frequency Monitoring System which is able to measure the electrical vibrational frequency of humans. He claimed that a healthy body resonates at 62–78 MHz, but disease can begin to take hold once the body drops to 58 MHz or below.[14]

Human Frequency Chart

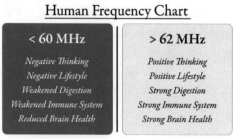

< 60 MHz	> 62 MHz
Negative Thinking	*Positive Thinking*
Negative Lifestyle	*Positive Lifestyle*
Weakened Digestion	*Strong Digestion*
Weakened Immune System	*Strong Immune System*
Reduced Brain Health	*Strong Brain Health*

Human bodies work best between 62 and 72 MHz

The idea of using frequency for healing is not new. Dr. Hulda Clark, a naturopath with a PhD in physiology, considered her books on this subject to be her gift to humanity. Dr. Clark spent much of her time helping to develop the research of Royal Raymond Rife, MD. In the 1920s, Dr. Rife developed a "frequency generator," the Rife Device.

In his research, he showed that certain frequencies enhanced health by destroying parasites, viruses, bacteria, and cancer cells—and that, by using his Rife Device, it was possible to prevent illness by improving the immune system. Proponents of the Rife Device, which delivers low-energy electromagnetic frequency into the body and is still available today, applaud its successful use as a treatment for pain; many suggest that the technique can be effective against some forms of cancer and some viral and bacterial diseases. The technique is based on the concept that every disease has its own electromagnetic frequency. Studies have shown that low-frequency waves affect cancer cells and normal cells differently, but research is ongoing, and critics deny that there is conclusive evidence of any benefit. Despite some evidence that low-energy waves kill cancer cells, more research is needed.

In her own research, Dr. Clark focused on environmental toxins as well as parasites. She went on to develop her own device, known as "the Zapper." She determined that frequencies between 290,000 Hz to 470,000 Hz were most effective at eliminating parasites. In this way, she pioneered the concept of "frequency-based-medicine."[15][16][17] She postulated that pollutants and parasites accumulate in the body and can be detected by the resonance of their frequencies using a device called a synchrometer. Although labeled a quack for some of her theories, Dr. Clark's "Zapper" device is seen by some as a health treatment breakthrough. Quantum frequency healing refers to the bio-electrical aspects of health and wellness. Using the principles of quantum physics, this method identifies and matches the frequencies of symptoms in order to support better health. This has been used for various ailments, from chronic pain and migraine relief to addressing depression and anxiety.

For the past twenty-five years, I have personally experienced the benefits of the Zapper. When anyone in my family feels unwell, they know to use the Zapper, and they have noticed that it helps shorten the length and severity of colds and flu. We also recognize that we are less contagious when we use this device. Today, there are new technologies emerging which are based on frequency through sound and light healing.

Imagination, Thought Forms, Beliefs, and Neuroplasticity

Creating anything always starts with an idea, a thought, an intention. In this way, we can agree that thoughts are powerful. Thoughts are forms of pure energy, or as mentioned, scalar waves. "Thought forms" are made up of many connected thoughts. They have a vibration that transmits information to our electromagnetic field. This information may seem to be positive or negative in nature and may be connected to our emotions and memories from our life stories and experiences.

As we grow in consciousness, we become more aware of our thoughts. We become the observer. We can follow the trails of our thought forms to our beliefs. Moreover, we can learn to control our thoughts and work with our beliefs to create *intentions*.

The exciting realization is that the universe is abundant; and as we use our imagination, the sky is the limit. Because we have, through consciousness, the ability to access the infinite resources of the quantum field, we also have the ability to create whatever we dare to think and dream about. As we see things more holistically and with fewer feelings of judgment and separation, we gain awareness that we are connected to everything. By being connected to all that is, we can start to use our imagination and create thoughts that serve our higher purpose. This empowers us to become more effective Creators.

Here is an example. Every six months, I market my course. First, I visualize the number of students I want to participate. I "see" them registering for the course, and affirm to myself, "I attract the right students easily." I then *feel* this statement as though it has already happened. When I first marketed the course, however, it was not this easy. I was often overwhelmed with fear, which would cause me to self-sabotage my efforts. In the end, I would always attract the right students and had enough money to pay the bills, but not before a long period of self-doubt and anxiety as I faced my fear of failure. (As I shared in Chapter Two, I'm an Enneagram Type 3, and this process of overcoming my fear of failure has been with me my whole life.) One spiritual teacher summed it up like this: some fears are lifetime-themed fears written on your template in pen. Each time you work on releasing them, you take an eraser to the ink, and it becomes a little bit lighter. The universe will continually test you by sending you new challenges to overcome, and eventually the ink will be erased forever.

BELIEFS, WORDS, AND ENERGY

Beliefs are often associated with particular themes, values, and areas of life. One belief can be linked to several other beliefs, and these collectively affect our decisions, behaviors, and life paths. These groupings of beliefs are called "belief systems."

We develop habits and patterns of behavior around our belief systems. We also express these ideas through the words that we choose. When I started to become more conscious, I became aware of all the words I chose when expressing myself. I started to notice connections between my words and my unconscious feelings about myself and the world. I also became aware of how the negative expressions I was using affected my creations. For example, I realized that I was often saying, "Life is crazy." The more I said this, the more I noticed how "crazy" life seemed. I consciously stopped saying this and instead opened myself up to using more positive expressions like, "Life is full of miracles." Once I made this change, I noticed that it became easier to manifest what I truly desired.

Psychology Dictionary defines a belief system as, "A set of beliefs which guide and govern a person's attitude. Usually, it is directed toward a system such as a religion, philosophy, or ideology. Attitudes and beliefs in these systems are closely associated with one another and retained in memory ... Your belief system is a set of attitudes and beliefs which mutually support each other for much of your life."[18]

Buddha took the power of belief one step further, saying, "All that we are is the result of what we have thought. The mind is everything. What we think, we become."[19] We create from our thoughts. Our thoughts influence our words and are linked to emotions. Basically, we create from what we *allow*. Part of the work of becoming conscious is learning how to manage our thoughts, feelings, and words so that we create the reality we desire, and not its opposite.

While this knowledge is ancient, neuroscience—the area of science that deals with the structure and function of the brain and nervous system— is now proving the power of our thoughts and beliefs. As it turns out, our thoughts and emotions are connected via our neural networks. They form neural pathways which develop uniquely based on our individual experiences and perceptions.[20]

When we are young, we have many connections. As we grow and develop in the first three years of life, we go through a process called "synaptic pruning," where we uniquely prune away connections that do not define us or our experiences any longer. Synapses are the connections between neurons. We transmit information through chemicals like neurotransmitters between our neurons. As we learn more information, certain synapses get stronger, and we also establish new pathways; this process is called neurogenesis. As we grow up, we prune and define our pathways to become our unique selves. As we age, we must continue this synaptic pruning in a more conscious way as a sort of neural "spring cleaning" so we don't unconsciously carry around beliefs and thought forms from earlier in our lives that no longer serve us or are causing congestion in our energy field.

This is where neuroplasticity comes in.

Neuroplasticity is defined as "the brain's ability to reorganize itself by forming new neural connections throughout life."[21] We can literally change our mind. How we take care of ourselves must therefore include observing, assessing, and pruning the thoughts we allow, the feelings we feel, and the toxins we ingest at all levels of our being. This, along with taking care of our physical bodies, will make a difference in how our brain ages, but also how it serves us in the here and now.

Each of our thoughts has a frequency. So do the words we say. Both of these are rooted in our beliefs. The beliefs we choose to carry or prune, the thoughts we allow, the emotions those thoughts generate, and the words we say will influence our future selves through neuroplasticity. Every day, we are literally teaching ourselves who we will become in the future.

Emotions and Frequency

Our thoughts and self-talk influence which emotions may be triggered from both our conscious and unconscious states. Emotions have frequencies (low to high) that impact our electromagnetic field on all levels. In duality, we have had the intense experience of feeling the lowest (guilt, apathy, grief, and fear) in opposition to the highest (love, joy, peace, and enlightenment). These lower emotions help us to survive. They also help us understand and manage duality. As we transition out of duality, we will begin to have more freedom to choose what frequency we will hang out in. As we ascend, we will begin to live from higher and higher emotional states without the need to experience lower-frequency emotions.

The Emotional Guidance Scale, shown below, is derived from the work of Dr. David Hawkins, and shows the frequency associated with each emotion.

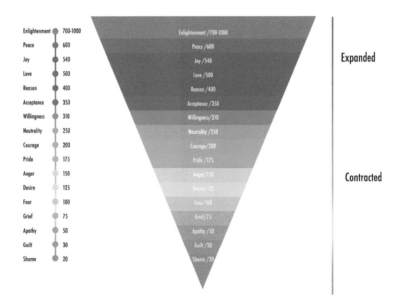

As we become more conscious and begin to understand that we create our reality, we may ask, "How do emotions fit into my stories and beliefs?"

We know that when we feel a high-frequency and powerful emotion, we feel uplifted by an energetic flow of expansion. On the other hand, when we feel a negative emotion, our energy begins to contract, and we can feel stuck, heavy, or closed-off. Over time, as we ignore these negative emotions, our bodies may become affected; we can begin to feel tired, depleted, and unhappy.

Two things are certain. One: emotions can be tremendously powerful, regardless of where they are on the frequency spectrum. Two: as we grow in consciousness and become the observer, we will begin to tune into how our emotions are connected to our stories and beliefs, and to what our emotions are actually trying to tell us.

Emotions are *messages.* They exist to guide us, much like a compass does. They show us how we are doing within our stories. If we feel a positive emotion, we are most likely going in the right direction. If we feel a negative emotion, we are most likely experiencing something in our life story that needs to be looked at.

Now, let's be clear: emotions and feelings are not the same. Emotions are the raw frequencies that happen within our bodies. Feelings are the links to the thoughts, emotions, and beliefs surrounding our stories; they are how we interpret our emotions within the context of our personal stories. As we grow and pay attention to how we feel, we can learn to manage our emotions and feelings and release any emotional baggage we are carrying. By accepting our emotions and feelings, we can digest and then release them.

Our emotions have a significant influence on the health of our electromagnetic field. Increasingly, medical science is acknowledging that much about people's health is determined by the state of their emotions. When you realize how many prescriptions are written for mood altering and elevating drugs—including hormones—you'll realize that it cannot be otherwise. Estrogen and testosterone are common sex hormones known to influence emotions and behavior. Dopamine and serotonin are known as reward and happiness hormones, and their workings in the brain have been extensively studied. Neuroscience is constantly busy with analysis of what hormones are related to which emotions, and both the pharmaceutical industry and illegal drug manufacturers are constantly on the lookout for chemicals to induce feelings of joy and wellness.

While drugs can be a lifesaver for many, they are only a temporary fix. Until we digest the emotions and stories we have been avoiding, they cannot fully correct the problem and bring us into a new level of Creatorship.

Fear and stress can lower our vibration; there is evidence linking suppressed anger to the development of cancer.[22] Many studies encourage cancer patients to work on anger management issues in their healing journey from cancer. As mentioned earlier in this chapter, Masaru Emoto's experiments show that loving and compassionate thoughts and emotions, like gratitude and joy, change the molecular structure of water, making it clear, brilliant, and crystalline. In contrast, water exposed to negative thoughts and lower-frequency emotions, like anger and sadness, took on a structure that was chaotic. If our bodies are composed of 70 to 80 percent water, and water is influenced by thoughts, words, and emotions, we then have tremendous creative power over how our mind, body, and spirit will function, and at what frequency they vibrate, and choose the emotional state that we elect to hang out in. People know that they are "masters" when they have conquered this ability; no matter what happens to them, they are able to remain neutral and in gratitude.

Quantum science underlines this concept. Many current studies have shown that our thoughts are electric, and our emotions are magnetic. These thoughts and emotions together influence our bio-individual electromagnetic field, which in turn interacts with the quantum field to create our physical reality.

With the power of digestion and our ability to consciously identify and change our stories and beliefs, we can learn to move in and out of emotions more quickly. It's no coincidence that our digestive system—which corresponds to our second and third chakras—is also our emotional processing center! When we can harness the power of digestion, we will always have a choice as to which emotional states we hang on to, and which we let go.

EMOTIONS AS PART OF OUR BIO-INDIVIDUALITY

Our emotions are another aspect of our bio-individual health as humans. We all have emotions, but most of us are not taught how to manage them. As we grow in consciousness, we realize that in order to be balanced and happy we need to manage our emotions.

As described above, emotions are what happen in the body, while feelings are how we interpret those emotions. Through our feelings, emotions help us connect to our experience. They let us know how we are doing. They let us know whether we feel safe or not via a feedback loop of feeling pleasure or pain. Pain, by its very nature, gives us a very uncomfortable feeling, and pleasure helps us feel joy, bliss, and even ecstasy.

Our emotional brain works with both the frontal cortex and the amygdala (limbic system). Feelings of happiness and pleasure are often linked to our frontal cortex, while feelings of anger, fear, and sadness happen in the amygdala. As mentioned earlier, our amygdala is constantly scanning our environment, trying to determine whether we are safe or not, and what responses and behaviors we require for survival. The frontal cortex also helps to regulate our emotions, either positively or negatively, especially with regards to our relationships and our social environment. As mentioned previously, we make decisions and control our emotional responses through the frontal cortex, but when we feel unsafe, the amygdala takes over, activating our "fight, flight, or freeze" response. This stimulates our adrenal glands to release cortisol—aka, the stress hormone. We might sweat or feel our heart pounding as adrenaline is released.[23] In this way, emotions are expressed through hormones.

Our emotions are also related to our facial expressions, which is why it is often easier to read the emotions of others than it is to recognize our own. As we grow in consciousness, we become more aware of our own emotions and reactions, and also about how others view us. As a child in our large family, I felt very sensitive to criticism as I experienced it as a form of rejection. Yet, as I have helped people heal over the years and gone through my own process of digestion, I am now far less afraid of self-reflection and criticism.

Emotion at the Cellular Level

The influence of emotions at the cellular level has been studied by Candice Pert. Remember that thoughts are electric and connect to emotions that are linked to a magnetic wave. In her book, *Molecules of Emotion,* she describes how emotions impact our health at the cellular level. Our emotions are communicated throughout our bodies via signals that connect at the cell membrane. Her studies led her to conclude that emotions are the link between the physical and the non-physical, and that this linkage happens at the receptors on every cell. Her contention is that the mind and body can't be treated separately, as done for example by physicians and psychologists, because they are not separate but intricately interlinked. This is confirmed by the chemical fingerprints of emotions as registered by hormones in the blood and brain.[24]

Through her research, Pert found that the cell membrane was, in fact, the brain of the cell. There are receptors sitting on the cell membrane that conduct the frequencies for communication. This was revolutionary because mainstream science has believed for a century that the nucleus is the "brain" of the cell.

The cell receptors float on the membrane, and in this way are the connection between the emotion being transmitted and the tissue. Pert writes: "A receptor vibrates and hums as it changes shape, waiting to pick up messages that diffuse through the fluids surrounding the cells.

A *ligand* is the chemical key that fits in the receptor, in a process called "binding" and "binding is sex on a molecular level."[25] This means that emotions trigger a physical molecule in the form of a hormone called a neuropeptide ligand to be released.[26] These ligands relay information via frequencies to the receptors and in this way give instructions to the cell to elicit a specific behavior. The receptors on our cells act like connections or docking stations for these "molecules" of emotion (neuropeptide ligands). When a person feels an emotion, the brain conducts information through a series of cell signals, sending hormones to these docking receptors in all cells of our body. Receptors cover all cells of our body and act like sensors or scanners. They can be compared to our senses (ears, eyes, nose, and skin, for example). We will learn more about these receptors when we study the new field of glycoscience in Chapter Nine.

What is important to understand is the power emotions have on us. If you are feeling joy, peace, courage, and love, this frequency will dock on your cells. On the other hand, if you are feeling fear, guilt, shame, or sadness, *these* frequencies will dock on your cells. Your emotions matter. We can therefore become addicted to a particular neuropeptide and the cyclic pattern it produces. This set of ligand responses can be as addictive as an opiate receptor. As mentioned in Chapter Four, in the long run these lower frequency emotions that are grounded in fear can set off a cascade of hormonal responses that can lead to stress-related diseases. For example, if a person has a thought of being unworthy that connects to a feeling of sadness, the molecule of emotion that transmits the feeling of sadness (in the form of hormones) will dock on all cells of the body with that information. In this way, our bodies are transmitting different emotions, which have different frequencies, all day long.

This is how, when we tune into someone's emotional state, we can pick up on their emotions—or, more accurately, their emotional frequency. Each of our human cells also has an electromagnetic field that transmits the frequencies of our thoughts and emotions. We can and will learn to read these emotions very accurately as we grow in consciousness. Some people call this "gut instinct," while others call it "reading energy." Depending on which of your seven ethereal senses are strongest, you may read emotional energy differently than others. We can all do this; some of us have simply developed or nurtured this ability more than others.

Pert also believes that memories—in the form of repressed emotions buried in the unconscious mind—can be stored and become stuck at the cellular level. Some of these emotional experiences are traumas and can dramatically influence our responses and behavior. Throughout our days, most of us can transition and process our emotions. However, if something happens that is particularly negative, it becomes more challenging to digest, and emotions can then get stuck. In this way, they can affect our mood, biochemistry, behavior, and health.

It seems complex, but we can absolutely influence how our emotions affect us on a cellular level. As we become more conscious, work with our stories and beliefs, and learn to manage our emotions, we learn to discern what is worth reacting to and what is simply lowering our frequency. If emotions are important indicators of how we are navigating our life, then discerning which emotions we allow to influence us is part of this. Most of us can relate to the following story. When we wake up, we are all excited to begin a new day. We are hopeful for what this new day will bring. The phone suddenly rings, disrupting this peace with news that the car, which had broken down a few days prior, will be costly to repair. We think about all the extra expenses of the past month and groan. Then, we turn on the news, only to hear that the stock market has crashed and war has broken out overseas. At this point, our mood has changed; we feel anxious, and the excitement and joy we felt earlier that morning has completely gone. An interesting question could be, why do we allow news or (relatively) minor challenges to alter our reality?

Emotions are an invitation to experience this earthly life deeply and more intensely. Imagine a life here on Planet Earth without emotions. What would that be like? Emotions connect us with the very essence of who we are and wish to be. They also help us to connect with others, and act as a compass when we make decisions. We can choose which emotions we decide to befriend and which we learn to pass through.

Learning that we have a choice in how we interact with our emotions gives us freedom. Although most of us are unaware of this, we can become addicted to emotional dramas in our lives. In truth, emotions can be compared to water. Feelings can connect us to the depths of our soul; and like water, we can release them by feeling them, accepting them, and letting them go—or, shall I say, flow! While it is not always easy to flow with and befriend our emotions, especially if the storyline surrounding it has not been accepted and digested, we must embrace this as part of our practice of Creatorship.

Changing Your Relationship to Energy

We are Creators—and, as we've discovered in this chapter, the frequency of our thoughts, words, and emotions influence what we manifest into matter. Our electromagnetic field has a dominant frequency that is directed by us. Understanding this concept will help us comprehend the magnitude of our creative ability. Plasma forms into specific geometric patterns depending on the messages we have given it; however, it does not seem to matter if we have done this consciously or unconsciously. As we become increasingly conscious of what we allow ourselves to think and feel, we will begin to see changes in what is manifesting on a physical level for us.

To realize that we influence the unseen world, we must become conscious that it exists. Many, as they wake up to this realization, begin the process by taking better physical care of their bodies. Others connect to their spiritual energy fields, while still others work on changing mental and emotional processes. What I have found is that it doesn't really matter where we begin. What matters is simply starting the process of observation and growing our awareness. Learning that what we allow and focus on impacts our destiny is a critical aspect of our evolutionary development and the effective management of our Creator Matrix.

Chapter Summary

- We humans *are* energy beings having a temporary stay in a human body to have experiences that allow us to connect to, manage, and master our electromagnetic energy field.

- The science of quantum mechanics explains how the universe works on a subatomic level, with focus on the behaviors of matter and light. Plasma makes up as much as 99 percent of all matter.

- Sacred geometry looks at the blueprint of matter, it looks at how the fundamental structures are organized. Structure is function. The universe is intelligent and has self-organizing mechanisms that act as a template for all creation.

- Within our body we have an energy system in which life force energy—chi, qi, ki, or prana—flows through energy meridians and seven energy portals or chakras which connect to Universal Source energy. It is important to keep our energetic system vital, flowing and free of blockages.

- The Law of Attraction is closely related to the Law of Vibration. Our thoughts and feelings influence our vibration and frequency, which influences our electromagnetic field. Our field influences what we attract into our reality and how it manifests, since like attracts like.

- The Law of Vibration is based on the principle that nothing rests, everything moves and is always in motion. When the energy of the body is able to revitalize and restore, it is in motion and healthy. When the energy of the body is congested or blocked due to toxins, stress, or undigested emotions, to name but a few, the system cannot function efficiently and can lead to imbalance and disease.

- Energy and matter change form depending on their rate of frequency. To become matter, energy moves from pure spirit—the highest vibrational level—to a lower-density vibration.

- Everything has a frequency: our thoughts, emotions, physical bodies, viruses, bacteria, parasites, animals, even atoms. Our health is directly correlated with the frequency we have on all levels of our Creator Matrix. Frequency-based medicine is the concept of using frequency for healing.

- Neuroscience—the area of science that deals with the structure and function of the brain and nervous system— is now proving the power of our thoughts and beliefs. Our thoughts and emotions are connected via our neural network, forming unique neural pathways, based on our individual experiences and perceptions. Loving self-care includes learning how to observe and consciously choose which beliefs we will focus on.

- Our thoughts, emotions, belief systems, words, and attitudes are composed of energy and influence the field and what we manifest.

- Emotions are messages to guide us, they are connected to our stories and beliefs, and they have frequencies that impact our electromagnetic field. By accepting our emotions and feelings, we can digest, release them, and befriend them.

- Emotions are shown to influence our cellular health. Becoming conscious of the emotions we are feeling can help us release low-frequency emotional patterns, as emotions can be stored and become stuck at the cellular level and can affect our mood, biochemistry, behavior, and health.

Chapter Seven

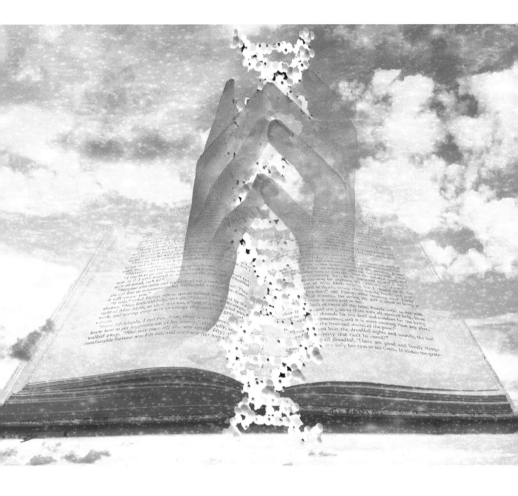

*How are your choices and your
storyline influencing your DNA?*

"Epigenetics suggests that we can signal our genes to rewrite our future."

- Dr. Joe Dispenza

CHAPTER SEVEN

Epigenetics

We have seen how we can heal ourselves from within by changing our stories, beliefs, and habits, and discovered the role consciousness plays in well-being and Creatorship. We have been focused on the power of the mind, emotions, and spirit. Now, we are about to take a deeper journey—a journey into the body to explore how the way we choose to live and the choices we make will make the difference in how we manifest physical health and well-being or illness. We will take a look at how many factors, including our lifestyle choices in general, can affect our DNA. Many people feel powerless to control what happens in their bodies. They think of their bodies as separate from their minds and consciousness, but that couldn't be further from the truth. The truth is, it *all* matters: how we handle our thoughts and emotions *and* how we care for our physical bodies will define how we age and the levels of happiness and fulfillment we can reach.

With more light on the planet, we can see more. Much is being disclosed and exposed. This whole awakening can make us feel uncomfortable. We are now being called upon to pay attention, reflect, participate, and persevere. We can no longer entrust our physical health solely to institutions or other people. Instead, we must increase our self-awareness and expand our consciousness so that we can govern and participate in self-directed healing.

We are awakening to the idea that our very DNA can change and be upgraded. It's up to us! We will repeat what we have not repaired or healed—and that includes what has not been healed within our DNA, cells, and tissues. We can choose to heal by releasing programs that no longer serve us. We are not completely helpless to determine what happens to us; rather, as we grow in consciousness, our very DNA can transcend its limited version and upgrade to an expanded potential. We can compare this to a computer system. As our systems become more complex and make more connections, the software quickens and becomes more efficient. We are familiar with the idea of upgrading our computers, so this can be a useful metaphor when looking at the body. As we discussed in Chapter Four, our bodies are like the hardware of a computer and our DNA is like the software. The new science of epigenetics is helping us understand that we are more influential than we realize when it comes to which genes are expressed and which are not.

Put more simply, science is showing us that what we think, feel, and do matters more than we ever knew.

Cause and Effect: The Roots of Imbalance and Disease

When I was working in the hospital, we were trained to look at illness through a limited lens. The nursing staff and doctors were mainly focused on treating and alleviating a patient's symptoms, not finding the root cause of the disease. Although alleviating others' suffering is compassionate and important, in my experience there was little time to work with patients on changing lifestyle behaviors. Nor were there enough resources to create an atmosphere for well-being in the hospital. Our treatment style often left patients feeling that there was very little they could do to change their situation except follow their doctor's orders and take the prescribed medication regime. Many of them left the hospital with the idea that they were fortunate if they were still alive in a few years; that their disease could be managed but not cured, and that they were stuck with their genetic fate.

Scientists at that time truly believed that human beings were victims of their genes. I remember asking one doctor if it mattered that I was eating a lot of sugar and carbohydrates. He replied, "No, your diet won't make a difference in alleviating the symptoms you are having in your gut. These gut issues probably run in your family." Although, on the one hand, I think he may have been correct, because I remember my mom suffering from irritable bowel syndrome (IBS), I was surprised that he did not ask me anything else about my lifestyle. My mother was a heavy smoker and drinker. We now know that these habits increase the chances of intestinal inflammation. Moreover, we know that too much sugar and carbohydrates in our diet can also contribute to gut inflammation.

What we do to, and with, our bodies matters. As we age, our body keeps a scorecard. We are either in balance, or we are not. Our bodies will eventually show us the reality of our choices by manifesting vibrant health or disease. Genetics is only one part of the storyline, and science is proving that our own behavior and the environment that we live in are far more powerful contributors to our well-being than our genetic predispositions.

As mentioned in Chapter Four in the discussion about disconnection, to understand disease we need to understand that the body is "not at ease." When we are unwell, it is because something within the body, mind, and spirit matrix is no longer functioning optimally. All these dimensions need to be connected and flowing as one unit for someone to feel well.

Many factors can contribute to imbalance. How we feed, clean, react to, and love our bodies will determine much of what happens to them. For example, we are learning that diet/nutrition and detoxification are the most important actions at the physical level to maintain cellular well-being. Our bodies build structures every day that are essential for cellular function, and we need to clean up toxins to allow our cells to rest, repair, grow, and die. When something goes awry, we need to give the body time to repair and heal. Keeping in mind that we make a million cells a second, imagine how much support our body needs in order to be able to carry out the tasks of growth, repair, healing, and rejuvenation each and every day.

Sleep plays a vital part in this process. It allows our body, mind, and spirit complex time to rest and digest. How we move and exercise the body is also very important. If we don't use it, we will lose it. When we don't allow ourselves enough sleep, or when we stop moving, we begin to feel out of balance. We start to become more toxic and overwhelmed. We may have trouble dealing with any added stress. The body may start to communicate this by waking up tired, having frequent headaches, and feeling anxious and depressed, just to name a few possible consequences.

In my experience taking health histories from patients and clients, I am often struck by the fact that a person's "imbalanced state" has become their "normal state," and they are simply living in perpetual survival mode—at least, up until a final stressor or trigger occurs. An accident or injury, a separation or divorce, the death of a loved one, financial problems, or other sudden traumas are often the catalysts that push patients over the edge and into a state of disease. Sometimes, the patient is not even aware of this final stressor as a trigger because their life has been feeling difficult for some time. Thriving is not in their consciousness.

Perception and self-care matter in the mastery of our earthly life. It is impossible to care for oneself when there is no space or intention for it. I often found that the underlying reason for this is a lack of worthiness and self-love. The opposite is also true. A strong, loving sense of self and a supportive family and social network have shown to support more positive outcomes; even if the patient eventually passes away, they do so with greater peace and ease knowing they are loved, cherished, and supported.

Epigenetics: Above Genetics

We cannot be balanced and well without our cells being balanced and well. Our body, mind, and spirit complex is connected to and influences the fate of every cell in our body. Epigenetics is the branch of research that looks at this connection and influence.

Conrad Waddington, a biologist and geneticist, coined the term "epigenetic landscape" in 1957 as a metaphor to describe how cells are influenced in a particular direction just like marbles rolling down a hilly landscape. As the landscape develops, so too does a certain irreversibility of each marble's direction, as each will always seek to roll to the lowest point. By changing how the landscape develops, the path of cell development and genetic expression can also be altered. The Embryo Project described it thusly: "The epigenetic landscape is a visualization of the interaction between genes and the environment by modeling the developmental pathways a cell can take during differentiation."[1]

Of course, in 1957, we had not yet begun to understand DNA, nor had we mapped the human genome. Still, Waddington's assessment holds true. Today, epigenetics can be defined as "the study of the biological mechanisms that switch genes on and off [and] how these genes are read in each cell of our bodies."[2] The word *epigenetics* literally translates to "above genetics."

Epigenetics teaches us that when we change the landscape, we change the outcome. Many health challenges that we once thought were beyond our power to influence are, in fact, both preventable and reversible. Just like we can alter the landscape of our minds by changing our beliefs, thought forms, and stories, we can influence the landscape of our bodies through our emotions, habits, and lifestyle choices. As we learned in earlier chapters, the body, mind, and spirit are inextricably connected via our Creator Matrix; what changes one will change the others, and what heals one will heal the others.

In my work in hospitals, I have witnessed spontaneous healings and remissions that some referred to as "miracles." Doctors were at a loss for words. No one could explain these sudden transformations. In my view, epigenetics played a part in these healings; when the emotional and spiritual landscape of the patient shifted, so too did the person's physical reality. Similarly, when the physical landscape changes, the emotional and spiritual aspects can also shift.

When I was younger, I was taught that our genes were the most important determining factor for our health. To me, this meant that whatever I did to take care of my body (or not take care of it) would not matter. If I was born with a cancer gene, I would probably get cancer. If I was born with a diabetes gene, I would probably get diabetes. You got what you got, and you just had to live with it. This took my power away and left me feeling fearful, powerless, and like a victim of my genetic lineage.

Epigenetics tells a much different story. For example, anxiety and stress-related disorders are common across the globe. Often, it is assumed that our genes for mental health are inherited, and that if our parents or grandparents suffered from mental health challenges, so too will we. Although there is a genetic component to nearly all diseases, the question is not whether the associated genes are present, but instead, whether they are *expressed* (either turned on or turned off)—and the answer to which genes get expressed is far more complex.

Unsurprisingly, one of the key determinants of gene expression is stress.

Research is only now beginning to show us the full scope of the negative impact of stress on our cellular health. As we've learned, an overstimulated sympathetic nervous system sends signals to our adrenals to stimulate cortisol and blood flow from our brain to our arms and legs. This activates the "fight, flight, or freeze" response and all its attendant mechanisms. Over time, this constant stimulation makes us susceptible to many stress-related imbalances and illnesses, from burnout and adrenal fatigue to obesity, diabetes, and cancer. However, whether we have genetic predispositions to such conditions is only part of the picture. The determining factor in the fate of each of our cells, and which genes within the cell are expressed, seems to be what we *allow* on all levels of body, mind, and spirit, and how we digest and integrate our experiences and emotions. Therefore, if we learn to manage our stress, nurture ourselves through our primary and secondary food choices, and proactively choose what we allow on all levels, we can have a powerful influence on our gene expression that supersedes our genetic inheritance.

To illustrate this more deeply we can look at the cell and its influences. When we change the landscape of our choices and the environment of the cell, we now understand that this can affect cell behavior. The traditional teachings of genetics taught us that the control center or "brain" of the cell was the nucleus. However, we have learned from Candace Pert that our emotions affect our cell membrane (Chapter Six). We will also discuss more about this in the chapter on glycoscience (Chapter Nine). As Dr. Bruce Lipton explains in his research, a cell can live with its nucleus removed for two months or longer. This means that what happens at the cell membrane level matters and will influence the fate of the cells.[3] You can compare epigenetics to the making of a movie: our genetic profile is the initial script, and our cells are like actors playing their roles. The script only gives us the initial instructions we, as the "directors" of our stories, influence what happens at the cellular level. We can focus on certain actions, rewrite the dialogue, and even eliminate certain scenes in pursuit of the final cinematic vision. Even though the director seems to be behind the scenes, their choices, their instructions, and even their moods are what ultimately create the final product. We can conclude that how we care for our Creator Matrix will have a large impact on our genetic expression, with the consequence of health or disease.

In other words, who we choose to become creates the conditions for health and wellness, and also for illness. As Dr. Lipton explains in his published research, our thoughts, feelings, and intentions can influence our DNA.[4] The HeartMath Institute has shown that feelings like love, appreciation, anger, and anxiety can influence genetic outcomes as powerfully as lifestyle habits like diet, smoking, and alcohol use.[5]

When it comes to our physical bodies, we have far more power as Creators than we have ever known or understood. Even if we have not made the best choices in the past, we have the power to change our behaviors in the now moment. Like building a sandcastle and knocking it down, we have endless opportunities to revisit the ways in which we are supporting our well-being.

Epigenetics and the Epigenome

When looking at risk factors for disease, medical researchers study environmental influences as well as personal choice influences. Risk factors for heart disease, for example, are family history, but also smoking, alcohol use, dietary factors, obesity, high blood pressure, stress, and/or limited exercise. Most of those factors come down to our lifestyle choices.

Epigenetics is the study of how behaviors and environment can cause changes that affect the way genes work. Epigenetics refers to all the factors that influence genetic outcomes. These can be factors coming from one's environment like stress, pollution, radiation, medicines, drugs, alcohol, chemicals, bacteria, and viruses, but also other environmental influences like social contacts, family interactions, and intimate relationships. The epigenome is further influenced by our food/nutrient intake, weight management, exercise regime, sleep routines, limiting beliefs, and emotional reactions. In a study entitled, "Changes in Prostate Gene Expression in Men Undergoing an Intensive Nutrition and Lifestyle Intervention," researchers found that changing lifestyle habits can change gene expression. By changing certain lifestyle habits, over 500 genes in the study subjects were either upregulated or downregulated.[6] This shows us that certain genes that promote wellness were turned on due to lifestyle and nutritional changes, while genes promoting illness were turned off.

Our choices, we now know, play a role in how we age, what frequency we vibrate at, and ultimately how our genes are expressed in different kinds of cells. The higher we keep our overall frequency, the healthier we will stay.

How does this work? Scientists have been discovering what the

DNA sequencing means, what is normal, and which sequences are linked with inherited diseases. Epigenetic influences do not change your DNA sequence like genetics can, but they can change how, where, and when your body *reads* a DNA sequence. The double helix is wrapped around proteins, and these can regulate whether a gene is turned on and off. The epigenome is the structure of proteins and chemical compounds that can connect to the DNA and tell the genome what to do. The epigenome is involved in the development of many common diseases like cancer, autoimmune, heart disease, and immune function.

When epigenetic compounds attach to DNA, they can change its function. In this way epigeneticists refer to this as "marking" the genome. These "marks" or "tags" change the way cells use the DNA's instructions. DNA is like a vast library with many books and the epigenetic influence will determine how, where, and when they will be read and used. The epigenetic marks can be passed between cells and sometimes passed on through generations. Nutrigenetics and nutrigenomics are subcategories of epigenetics. They look at the dietary response, the role of food/nutrients, and the lack thereof in gene expression. We will look at this further in Chapter Eight.

You might ask: how exactly does this epigenetic mechanism work? For instance, what is the role of our epigenome in developing cancer? Cells grow and differentiate by the instructions given by the epigenome. All cells specialize with different functions depending on where they are in the body.

One aspect of epigenetics is looking at DNA methylation. This is a process by which cells are blocked from activation or activated to express some action in the body. Methyl groups or tags are added to the DNA molecules in specific places for specific tasks. These methyl groups turn genes on and off. Methylation is when the genes are turned on, and demethylation is when the genes are turned off.

Methylation is responsible for many cellular activities. When DNA methylation is abnormal or disrupted, then disease can occur. As we age, many scientists believe that DNA methylation slows down and genes that were previously repressed can become active. When these chemical groups or tags are added to these specific places on the DNA, the protein is blocked from reading the gene or instruction. When the chemical groups are removed, the proteins can then read the gene. So, getting back to how this process can influence us to develop cancer specifically; when methylation is abnormal due to toxicity (which can be caused by, among other things, a high intake of processed foods), certain genes like tumor suppressor genes can be silenced, and this can allow cancer cells to grow.[7]

Histones are another part of the epigenome story. Histones are proteins that DNA can wrap around. They keep the genome wrapped tight and organized. Histones can be marked as "open" or "closed," which allows the gene to be "on" or "off." When these histones are wrapped tightly around the DNA, the gene itself is in the "off" position and proteins cannot enter the DNA to read the gene. On the other hand, when the histones are wrapped loosely, proteins can gain access to DNA and read the gene. As chemical groups are added or removed from the histones, thus influencing them to be tighter or looser, the genes are turned on and off.[8]

Some common diseases can result from the failure of the proteins to both read and write the marks or tags. Once the gene is read, it is copied by messenger RNA to go to the ribosomes and make protein structures that will serve the needs of the cells and body at that moment. The clearer the message, the more efficient and precise the response by the body system. However, a breakdown in communication—for example, a wrong message sent or a misunderstanding of the message—can cause chaos in the system, and the final proteins may be made incorrectly and "misfolded." Misfolded proteins are responsible for many degenerative diseases like Alzheimer's, Parkinson's, and diabetes.

DNA can be either coded or non-coded. Coding DNA is used to make protein structures, whereas non-coding DNA is not involved in protein synthesis. Scientists used to call this non-coded DNA "junk DNA." The function of non-coding DNA is now better understood as scientists are questioning the very nature of DNA itself. Non-coded DNA has many influences on the function of cells and is directly involved in gene expression—both by regulating and sequencing the genes and also by influencing when and where genes are turned on and off.[9]

In conclusion, science is always evolving, much like we are. Ultimately, science is showing that epigenetics triumphs over genetics; our choices and ways of living directly impact the health and behavior of our cells, and this influences which genes we express and the overall health of our body systems.

Intentions and Emotions Affect Cellular Health and DNA Expression

As we have learned, mental, emotional, and spiritual influences can impact our health and well-being as much or more as physical influences. Studies have determined that negative close relationships are a key predictor of coronary disease. Women who were dissatisfied with their primary relationship were three times more likely to have metabolic syndrome. These findings were even more prominent among people living in deteriorated physical environments, such as impoverished neighborhoods. On the other hand, positive relationships with spouses, friends, and family seem to create "protective" factors that make people more resilient and less prone to disease.[10] What will become important moving forward is to find the connections between all these individual factors. We don't have to suffer. In fact, I've realized that one of the main purposes of our lives here on Earth is for us to connect with and experience love, joy, and happiness.

Working as a nurse, I saw firsthand that most people suffering from disease had one thing in common: they had become disconnected from their bodies, their emotions, their feelings, and ultimately, themselves as a Creator. It was as if some part of themselves had become completely separated from the whole and from who they really were. It did not seem to matter whether the person suffered from a mental imbalance, brain disorder, or an autoimmune/degenerative disorder; each person was being called, through the dis-ease in their body, to pay more attention to some aspect of themselves. For many, this realization brought their world to a complete halt. Part of them had stopped functioning optimally and was not connecting to the whole anymore.

As I shared in Chapter Four, this idea of disconnection and its correlation with dis-ease still bothered me even after I left nursing. This led me to my research about what transpires with emotions, thoughts, and stories at a cellular level. For there to be connection, there must also be communication between all the cells; like our thoughts, energy, and emotions, every cell in our bodies is part of our Creator Matrix. But if wellness means optimal cellular communication, what causes cellular disconnection? And could this cellular disconnection be blocking our connection to the Universal Field that governs all that is?

My research continued and I came to understand that toxicity was a major factor in this blockage. It was not only toxicity in the environment and in our food that contributed to this disconnection, but also emotional baggage and toxic thought patterns. Looking back, I understood that those patients who became well again had managed to reconnect with and heal the part of themselves that had become so out of balance.

In my life, whenever I feel unhappy or out of balance, physically, mentally, emotionally, or spiritually, I take the opportunity to reevaluate my path and how I am directing my life story. Every imbalance offers me the opportunity to reflect, digest, and potentially learn something new. As we become more aware and our consciousness grows, we can become more powerful in controlling our well-being at all levels by showing up as the Creator in our lives. Ultimately, we are able to integrate these parts of ourselves that have become disconnected. This process feels truly amazing.

One way to reconnect to our being is to connect to our heart. There is a connection between the heart's electromagnetic field (which is sixty times larger than that of the brain!) and the "sixth sense" or intuitive intelligence we explored in Chapter Five. Intuition is a very different phenomena than brain thoughts. It has been scientifically proven that when someone connects to the electromagnetic field of the heart and experiences a deep feeling of harmony, they can decrease their stress levels, increase productivity, and improve their health. This is especially true when combined with breathing techniques and positive emotions and affirmations.[11]

On a physical level, the heart has sensory neurons that communicate information directly with our brain as well as the rest of our mind, body, and spirit complex. This information helps us make sense of the world around us through our feelings and emotions. We can influence our ability to regulate our emotions and thought patterns by connecting the electromagnetic fields of both the brain and heart. A well-known quote by Alfred Adler states, "Follow your heart, but take your brain with you." This balanced feeling is often referred to as "heart coherence."

Connecting with the heart is also a way to connect to our soul. Practicing mindfulness and meditation helps to balance both the mind and heart. As we become more in alignment with our true selves, we will become clearer and more coherent. Although research on heart coherence is still in its infancy, I believe that it will change the course of humanity.

Masaru Emoto's work, which I introduced in Chapter Six, shows us that thoughts have an effect not only on what shows up in our reality, but also on the health and well-being of the cellular and molecular structures of our body. Moreover, Emoto's work shows that what we intend has power. Intention focuses our thoughts and makes them even stronger.

Emoto's work has been furthered by other researchers, like Lynne McTaggart, author of *The Intention Experiment*.[12] She has worked to create the "world's largest global laboratory on mass intention." Out of thirty-nine experiments conducted, she has managed to find evidence of thirty-five significant results.

Her first experiment was with psychologist Dr. Gary Schwartz, director of the Center for Advances in Consciousness and Health at the University of Arizona. In March 2007, a webcam was placed in front of a London audience with a live geranium leaf shown on it. There were two different leaves used. The audience was instructed to send an intention to one of the leaves for ten minutes in order to make it glow. However, they were asked to focus on one leaf only, not the other one. Both leaves were photographed by a digital CCD camera. The two leaves were inspected a week later. Dr. Schwartz found that, "the changes in the light emissions of the leaf given the glowing intention had been so strong that they could readily be seen in the digital images created by the CCD camera."

McTaggart's other experiments looked at how intention can change the structure of water. Since we, as humans, are made up primarily of water, our intentions may directly affect the structure of water, which is important for health. One of her studies was done after Dr. Emoto approached her with the idea to purify the polluted waters of Lake Biwa through intention. When looking at the structure of healing water, there are very different patterns than in polluted water. McTaggart conducted this particular experiment with Russian physicist Dr. Konstantin Korotkov of St. Petersburg State Technical University, who had previously done a great deal of research on many liquids, including water, using his own invention, the gas discharge visualization (GDV) technique. He discovered differences in blood samples between patients suffering from cancer or heart disease, as well as changes in water after it was irradiated. In this experiment, McTaggart and Dr. Korotkov asked both an online audience as well as a live audience to send the water within Lake Biwa an intention of love while holding in their minds an image of a mountain stream. In his report, Dr. Korotkov found that, "All presented results demonstrate that collective intentional mental influence has significant effect both on water parameters and on the condition of the space."[13]

McTaggart performed her first experiment on an actual person on April 26, 2014, and continues to expand her research to this day. She invites people to nominate someone weekly who needs healing and documents their amazing results on her website. Many miraculous results are published by those who have participated. Even people with extreme diseased states have reported healings.[14] These experiments have helped us to understand how our own consciousness affects what we manifest into our material reality.

Dr. Glen Rein, a cellular biologist, studied the effects of energy healing on biological systems. He asked the subjects to hold test tubes containing DNA while being healed. There were positive indicators that the DNA changed when exposed to these experiences. He then joined the HeartMath Institute, where he continued to study this correlation.

Still more researchers have looked at the influence our thoughts have on consciousness. They have studied the effects of our thoughts on water, our heartbeat, DNA,[15] EEG, and even on *random number generators (RNGs)*.[16] A study entitled "Modulation of DNA Conformation by Heart-Focused Intention" looked at heart rhythms in response to emotional states. They found that negative emotions like anger and worry made heart rhythms more irregular and disordered, while positive emotions like affection and kindness made heart rhythms more coherent and calmer. They concluded that people are able to alter or modulate their DNA through intentionality, especially when they are in a loving, heart-focused state.[17]

When we deliberately modulate our emotions, align our thoughts and intentions with our desires rather than our fears and dislikes, and control our reactions, we will begin to change not only our mental and emotional experiences but also our bodies themselves. This is when we truly become the Creator in our lives and refine our ability to manifest our deepest dreams and desires in physical form.

Recent breakthroughs in neuroscience indicate that our brains are constantly changing. They create and break down neural pathways all the time. When you do something often enough, the related neural pathways are strengthened. Every day, every second of every minute of every day, we are reshaping our brains anew. This creates possibilities for both positive and negative health and wellness outcomes.

As we learned in Chapter Four, "neuroplasticity" refers to the malleability of our neurons and neural pathways. The brain is constantly reorganizing itself and creating new neural connections with this process of neuroplasticity. This process enables neurons (nerve cells in the brain) to adjust to new activities (thoughts, emotions) and changes in the environment. As Dr. Joe Dispenza explains, "We are marvels of flexibility, adaptability, and a neuroplasticity that allows us to reformulate and repattern our neural connections to produce the kind of behaviors that we want."[18]

Every thought, behavior, and habit reinforces the strength of certain neural pathways. As we grow in consciousness, we discover that we have a choice as to which neural pathways we decide to strengthen. Reshaping our neural pathways does not happen overnight; research shows that it can take an average of twenty-one days at least, and often it can take months. The speed of the rewiring process depends on our motivation, our confidence, and our belief in our ability to change. However, both neuroscience and epigenetics confirm that change is not only possible, but also inevitable if the right process is followed.

Inherited Belief Systems and Our DNA expression

As we explored earlier in this book, each of us can carry belief systems, thought patterns, emotions, traumas, and storylines not only throughout our lives, but across generations and even incarnations. We have beliefs about everything—religion, money, power, other people, and ourselves, to name just a few. The thought forms, emotions, and neural programming of our parents, grandparents, and ancestors live on in our DNA. I have seen the results of carrying these outdated belief systems and emotions on my DNA through my own life stories. I began clearing my own blockages, as well as those of my family members, during my first years living in the Netherlands by working with José, the kinesiologist. She would ask my body, mind, and spirit complex where the blockages and distortions were coming from. As I developed my own coaching and holistic healing practice, I helped many of my clients recognize and reprogram imbalances that were imprinted at the cellular level. Almost all of them felt a difference after this process and described it as a "lightening up."

Many people never wake up to the fact that they may be carrying fears, beliefs, and attitudes that don't even belong to them. When we become more conscious of our limiting beliefs, we can get help to reprogram them. It is not necessary to always know where the blockages come from.

As I mentioned in Chapter One, I had some serious concerns about the health of my son when he was born, and this triggered many ingrained patterns in my body, mind, and spirit complex. I suffered from tremendous anxiety as a child, and it became more pronounced after his birth. What began as hypochondriacal worry quickly transformed into a postpartum anxiety disorder. I became obsessed with my concern for him and his health.

I went to José for help. She understood the severity of my worries and was eager to find answers for them. Through her Touch for Health method, she discovered that the worries I was having had been inherited from my great-great grandmother on my mother's side. I was shocked to discover from her that this ancestral relative had lost most of her children in some kind of epidemic. It seemed I had not only inherited my great-great-grandmother's rebellious spirit, but also her deep-seated fears and grief around the loss of her children. I was close to my grandmother and decided to verify the information I had received about *her* grandmother. I decided to call her, and I asked, "Mimi, can you tell me about your grandmother on your mother's side?" She immediately started to laugh and said, "Who, Mamma Alice? She was my favorite, and she also had a nervous disease. She and I had so much fun together until they put her in one of those loony places." She never got over losing so many of her kids; my mom was one of the few who survived."

My heart stopped in time as I was taken back to the session when José had found the emotion, beliefs, and trauma that I had inherited from Mamma Alice. At that moment of discovery, I almost couldn't breathe as I connected with Mamma Alice and this fear of losing my own children and my health. It became clear that both Mamma Alice and I didn't trust our bodies and felt tremendous anxiety and responsibility toward our children. She had the pain and grief of losing so many, and I carried these same fears in my very DNA.

I then reprogrammed my fears and emotions with José, who later became a dear colleague and friend. Letting go of the fear felt like a hundred-pound brick had been lifted from my soul. I left her office singing and crying, tremendously touched by how connected I felt to Mamma Alice. I noticed in the following weeks a lightness toward my son and his medical challenges. He healed very quickly after that, and our story changed. My preoccupation with his health and my own slowly became more balanced, and I could focus on my life's path again.

I continued to work with José to release fears and belief systems. Perhaps not surprisingly, I was continually brought back to that maternal family line. I had developed an imbalance of the thyroid. As a nurse, I understood the physical reasons for this, but now I was learning the importance of the emotions and thought forms behind it as well. It has always been important to me to be heard and taken seriously. I believed that my father had wanted me to be a boy. Although I was the eldest child, Dad seemed to connect more easily with one of my younger brothers who shared his love of sports and intellectual pursuits. Although I felt deeply loved by my father, I had trouble feeling as though he wanted to hear what I had to say. The emotions surrounding the feeling and belief system of "not being heard" left me struggling with frequent sore throats and general pain in the thyroid area. My father and I have since healed this and we can now laugh about it. I am grateful for him and our relationship as it has truly helped me love myself more deeply.

Once I left home and became a nurse, my story of "not being heard" continued with some of the doctors I worked with. When someone does not seem interested in what you have to say, a feeling of humiliation can arise. As I worked with José on this emotional blockage, I began to understand how powerfully this story had impacted my life. Again, she found a blockage on the same maternal line of DNA—and again, it originated with Mamma Alice.

As it turned out, this family line was very involved in the suffragette movement (as I mentioned in the Introduction). I now understood my mother and her political activism in a whole new way. I remembered my Mimi showing me photos of a suffragette, saying, "Don't ever forget how hard it was for women to get the right to vote. Always remember the power you have as a woman." My childhood self felt honored to have come from this lineage, but also unworthy of the way my fore-mothers had fought for my rights. Working with José, I was able to heal this sense of unworthiness and come to a sense of pride in my lineage and in my own worth as their beneficiary. After many years of working with José, I was able to heal and feel a freedom in myself.

I believe that all the clearing I have done has helped to change my gene expression. This may not be something I can literally prove (at least, not with current technologies), however I have experienced the physical changes of healing on all levels of body, mind, and spirit. I also have seen a difference in what storylines show up for both me and my family. On a physical level, I am free from the daily anxiety and panic attacks I used to suffer.

In order to illustrate the power of releasing ancestral blockages further, we can look at the fear of losing money, which is a fear I have helped many to release. I remember a grandfather who worked hard and had a thriving business, but in his ancestral line there was an ances-tor who was robbed and lost everything. No matter how hard Grandpa worked, something would happen, and he would lose all the money he had worked for. Someone would betray him, or he would simply lose it—on the subway, in a store, or through a bank error. Each time the situation happened, it reinforced his belief and fear that he would always lose his money.

When he became conscious of this pattern, it became important for this grandfather to change his subconscious limiting belief of lack and loss. He sought help from an NLP (Neuro Linguistic Programming) practitioner, who helped him change his belief of lack and loss and turn it into one of abundance and trust. Not only did this help the grand-father heal his money issues, but it also helped to heal the ancestral money issues for his children and grandchildren.

Creating Our Genetic Lineage

As you've seen in this chapter, epigenetics is showing us that everything we think, feel, perceive, nourish ourselves with, and choose in our lives affects which genes will be "turned on" and which will not. In this way we can change our DNA expression. Everything we do influences the fate of our cells. Our cells are constantly regenerating, thriving, or dying. As we grow in consciousness, we are becoming aware of these connections. Therefore, learning to live from our hearts and loving ourselves more completely will help us become more conscious of these influences, and may even help us choose more positive behaviors and habits to align our body, mind, and spirit matrix with this higher frequency. This is the work we must do to not only prevent disease, but also to heal our bodies. In this way, we take responsibility and become the Creator.

Chapter Summary

- Instead of trusting our physical health to institutions or other people, we must increase our self-awareness and expand our consciousness so we can govern and participate in self-directed healing.

- We are ascending. As we grow in consciousness, our DNA is transcending its limited version and upgrading to an expanded potential.

- Our body, mind, spirit complex is connected to and influences the fate of every cell of our body. Epigenetics looks at this connection and influence.

- Epigenetics means "above genetics" and looks at the interaction between genes and the environment. It studies the biological mechanisms that switch genes on and off and how genes are read in each cell of our bodies.

- When we change the environmental landscape, we change the outcome of cell development and alter the genetic expression.

- Science is showing that epigenetics triumphs over genetics and that our choices and way of living will directly impact the health and behavior of our cells, and this will influence which genes are expressed.

- Every cell in our body is part of our Creator Matrix. Toxicity on all levels, in the environment, in our food, emotional baggage, and toxic thought patterns are major factors in cellular disconnection and blocking our connection to the Universal Field that governs all that is.

- We can reconnect to our being and our soul by connecting to our heart. Heart coherence is the balanced feeling when the electromagnetic fields of both the heart and brain are connected. As we become more in alignment with our true selves, we will become clearer and more coherent. We feel better!

- Thoughts have an effect on what shows up in our reality and on the health and well-being of the cellular and molecular structures of our body. Intention focuses our thoughts and makes them even stronger.

- People are able to alter or modulate their DNA through intentionality, especially when they are in a loving, heart-focused state.

- When we deliberately modulate our emotions, align our thoughts and intentions with our desires (rather than our fears and dislikes) and control our reactions, we will begin to change not only our mental and emotional experiences but also our bodies themselves. This is when we truly become the Creator in our lives and refine our ability to manifest our deepest dreams and desires in physical form.

- Neuroscience shows that, via neuroplasticity, our brains are constantly changing, reorganizing itself, and creating new neural pathways. Our brain is flexible and adaptable to new activities and environmental changes.

- As we grow in consciousness, we discover that we have a choice as to which neural pathways to strengthen via consciously repeating choices of thoughts, behaviors, and habits over a period of time.

- In our DNA (epigenome) we can carry the inherited thought patterns, emotions, and neural programming of our parents, grandparents, and ancestors, which can influence our own life stories and gene expression. Therefore, it can be very powerful to release outdated beliefs and ancestral blockages for optimal health and wellness.

Chapter Eight

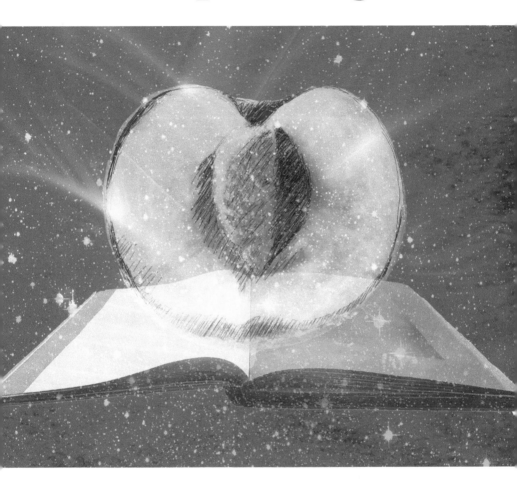

Food is information.
How are you nourishing your cells?

"When diet is wrong, medicine is of no use.
When diet is correct, medicine is of no need."

- Ayurvedic proverb

CHAPTER EIGHT

Nutrigenetics
and Nutrigenomics

Food has many different meanings for people. It often unites us, brings us into connection with each other, and helps us cope with and enjoy this earthly experience.

My father had a tremendous influence on my love of food. When he cooked his famous Italian meals, he always made them a celebration. It was a time to catch up, share, and unite with our large family and many friends. He still spends hours preparing special meals, and our family still looks forward to his delicious creations.

Each of us has our own traditions, preferences, and habits around food. We also have our own unique relationships with food and eating. Food can bring pleasure, and, as discussed earlier, the process of digesting and assimilating our food can help us digest our life stories and process our emotions. However, life can often feel out of control, and during those times food can become either a crutch or an enemy. During stressful times, some of us will eat everything in the fridge, while others cannot eat a single bite. When we begin to rely on food as our only source of happiness or pleasure, then this relationship has become dysfunctional and dependent.

One of the first things my clients begin to observe as they grow in consciousness is the food choices they make and their habits around eating. As they become more conscious of their relationship with food, they make different choices and begin changing the health trajectory of their life. Even clients with cancer have been able to recover and heal more quickly and easily by making more mindful decisions about what they eat. These types of food changes are often the first step toward becoming more conscious in all areas of life.

Nutrigenetics and Nutrigenomics

As discussed in Chapter Seven, our choices in all areas of life can influence our gene expression either positively or negatively. In this chapter, we will explore two more of the new sciences: nutrigenetics and nutrigenomics. Nutrigenetics looks at how people's genetics influence the ways in which their body will react or respond to certain foods, while nutrigenomics looks at the effect of food on gene expression. In this way, food is information.

Many people are struggling with their gut health at this time. Besides the emotional aspects of gut health we explored in earlier chapters, there is also a physical component. Early on in my life, I suffered a great deal from digestive issues, including constipation, and was later diagnosed with irritable bowel syndrome (IBS). I further learned how vulnerable my gut was when I took a trip to Brazil and was sick for almost a year with the parasite, *giardia*. While recuperating from this infection, I developed new, healthier habits, such as eating fewer processed foods, drinking less alcohol, and eating more fiber.

Later, when I was suffering from thyroid-related symptoms, I also tried an elimination diet. I eliminated "offending" foods like gluten, alcohol, genetically modified soy and corn, processed foods, and dairy for at least four weeks; after that, I reintroduced them one at a time at weekly intervals so I could evaluate the effects of each on my body. Before the elimination diet, I had been experiencing bloating, constipation, rashes after eating certain foods, fatigue, weight gain, low thyroid, and brain fog. Following the elimination diet, I noticed a definite improvement in my overall symptoms. Most of them disappeared, and I felt much better.

Since then, I've added other things into my diet that have really helped heal my gut lining, including healthy fiber, L-Glutamine, probiotics (good bacteria), and prebiotics like glycans (which I will discuss in depth in Chapter Nine).

When I was a nurse, it was not as clearly understood that diet influenced our ability to function optimally and feel good. Now, science is showing that what we eat matters because food is information. If we eat high-frequency, nutrient-dense foods, we will turn on and upregulate genes that promote growth, repair, detoxification, and health. If, on the other hand, we give our body food that has been altered, highly processed, or chemically preserved, it may block the genes that promote growth, repair, and detoxification, and instead stimulate genes that cause inflammation and disease.[1]

Many people are completely unconscious about how their food choices can change their gene expression and cause disease. Our modern way of living is often stressful and has a survival mode mindset. Many of us have a difficult time stepping off the hamster wheel and making the necessary time to change our habits and food choices. Understanding that food is information gives us the power to choose foods that serve us. And, since the very foods we choose will instruct and direct our genes to turn certain functions on and off, our choices can have powerful effects in both the short and long term.

Recent research is pointing to a new understanding of how this can happen. An article entitled "Ingested Plant MiRNAs Regulate Gene Expression in Animals" demonstrated the power of food on our gene expression. MicroRNA are non-coded RNA molecules found in some viruses, but also in plants and animals. When we eat plant or animal foods, these microRNA molecules are not broken down or altered; rather, they are transported through the gut to the bloodstream and into the cells, where they regulate and modify gene expression by transmitting information. In fact, the microRNA binds to the chromosomes, thus altering the outcome of that cell. In their analysis, the study's authors posed the question, "What is the potential consequence of genetically modified (GMO) microRNAs on our future gene expression and health?"[2] Given what we already know about the effects of GMO foods on the body, we can infer that those effects will not be positive.

PREVENTION IS NO LONGER ENOUGH

The first time I became part of the conversation about "prevention" was in college. I was studying Health Education, and everyone was talking about how to prevent illness. I thought this was a good idea—after all, who *wouldn't* want to stop themselves from getting sick?

In the medical community, many align prevention with early detection. Although this is important, it can also cause a great deal of unnecessary stress. How many people have had an early detection screening that showed abnormal cells or growths in their body that could not yet be diagnosed accurately, but which nevertheless prompted an extensive series of tests, scans, and fear-laden conversations? This kind of scenario happens more frequently than we realize. Unfortunately, there is little follow-up for patients who are not deemed to have "active" disease, and therefore little attention on helping them heal and rebalance.

In the medical community, "prevention" means "eat well and exercise to prevent disease." However, this is not enough to combat the challenges we are facing at this time. Remember, what we focus on expands. When you think about prevention, the logical next question is, "preventing what?" Immediately, your thoughts go to a particular disease or condition. However, given what we know about thoughts and emotions and their ability to influence our energy field, thinking about disease on a regular basis is not likely to be helpful in terms of our frequency and vibration.

This does not mean that we cannot try to avoid disease. On the contrary, the best way to begin to influence your body toward health is to focus on health! When we focus on what we are seeking rather than what we don't want, we are more likely to find it.

So, let me ask you: what does health look like for you? What does it feel like? If you want to practice prevention, spend time thinking and feeling "health and wellness" every day.

A Challenged Planet

As we evolve, we are waking up to the many challenges we are facing individually and collectively on our planet. The pathway for revolutionary wellness is emerging now as we are facing these challenges to our basic survival, both personally and globally. Apart from the many communicable diseases that threaten our species, a number of non-communicable diseases have reached alarming proportions. As the planet becomes more toxic every year, there are growing risks to human health that threaten the very survival of our species.

Through choices made with limited awareness by previous generations, children today are being brought up in a world full of environmental hazards. For example, a 2016 study by scientists at UC Berkeley and UC San Francisco found that blood in the umbilical cords of newborns contained some fifty-nine chemicals that didn't belong there.[3]

One of the most basic ingredients in health is the ability to breathe clean air. Literally billions of people live under polluted skies or cook over smoky open fires; compromised health is a predictable result. Millions more are forced to drink polluted or unsafe water contaminated by chemical residues from industrial processes and energy production. People are also taking all sorts of medications that are toxic to their bodies. Toxic habits like alcohol abuse, drug addiction, and smoking, to name just a few, should also be considered.

In conclusion, toxicity is one of the major issues challenging our cellular well-being and influencing the expression of our DNA. And, while it's tempting to blame previous generations and current institutions for the problems we are encountering, that is not ultimately helpful. Most people have done the best they could with the level of consciousness they possessed at the time. Rather, we must work together to seek out new solutions for both our individual health and that of the planet.

FOOD HAS BEEN ALTERED

As I have already mentioned several times, humanity has, before now, predominantly existed in a survival-based mentality. This way of thinking has created many limiting beliefs and fears, including with regard to our relationship with food.

Since we have always been creating our reality, even unconsciously, many of these fears laid the foundation for the timelines we are currently experiencing. One of these limiting beliefs is our deep fear of scarcity and malnutrition. Many of our decisions about food, both individually and collectively, have been based on the belief that there isn't enough for everybody, and that it is impossible for this planet to sustain us all. I always wondered what would happen if every person on the planet had another thought; namely, that the planet can produce and support more than enough food to sustain us. What if we had complete faith in the planet and ourselves to always create what was needed?

Today's commercial agriculture is the result of people looking for quick solutions to combat the problem of scarcity. This created new, more "efficient" ways of growing food. Unfortunately, many of these methods have not served us. We have, as a result of mass production and the commercialization of food, created a new problem: a preponderance of foods that are highly addictive but possess very little nutritional value. These foods are addictive and stimulate the same area of the brain that becomes aroused when someone uses cocaine—a "bliss point" that leaves us wanting more and more. Food marketing, especially of processed foods, has managed to get generations of consumers hooked on nutritionally empty foods, thus leaving them vulnerable to various diseases and health challenges.

What we eat is not only needed for daily energy, but also to build the structures of our cells themselves. We literally become what we eat at the cellular level. We are not like cars; we cannot simply "fill up the tank" with whatever fuel is at hand. Instead, we are building the "tank" each and every day with the foods we eat. If we fill it up with the incorrect fuel source, not only will the body not "drive" properly, but the tank itself will also be compromised. Keeping in mind that we make a million cells a second, we can see that eating foods that nourish us is critical for our health and wellness.

Many years ago, I had the honor of meeting a scientist named Larry Law, and his wife, Angie. They were teaching their Wellness Journey class. Larry knew a great deal about the new nutritional sciences. His wife, Angie, had been struggling for some time with her health and it was necessary for him to look beyond the obvious for answers. He taught me a great deal about the effects that a lack of good nutrition can have at the cellular level. In his book, *There's an Elephant in the Room: Exposing Hidden Truths in the Science of Health,* Larry writes, "The lack of real nutrition plays a dominant role in our health and well-being." He further explains that cancer is not only caused by "something," but by the "lack of something"—in particular, the lack of a normally functioning immune system to remain healthy.[4] Many people eating a modern diet are completely unaware of how much our food has been altered and how deficient it is in nutrition.

Good food, consisting of both macro- and micronutrients, is required to build healthy cells and keep "disease genes" from turning on. Eating more fresh vegetables and fruits helps create cells that function more optimally. Macronutrients are composed of the foods that provide fat, protein, and certain carbohydrates that create the proper structure for healthy cell functions. Micronutrients are the "helpers" like enzymes, vitamins, minerals, and antioxidants that make everything happen. The food industry has desperately tried to repair some of the damage caused by overprocessing by adding in certain missing nutrients; however, much of what is added is synthetic, and therefore less bioavailable for use in the body. Supplements, like all pharmaceuticals, are primarily synthetic, and many studies have shown the dangers of overusing synthetic medicines and supplements. In a 2016 study entitled "Vitamins, Are They Safe?" it was concluded that, "Taking [synthetic/non-organic] supplements of vitamin E, A, C, D, and folic acid for prevention of disease or cancer is not always effective, and can even be harmful to [the] health..."[5] Another study where synthetic beta-carotene and vitamin A were given to smokers and asbestos workers was halted due to alarming death rates, with deaths from lung cancer increasing by 46 percent and deaths from cardiovascular disease increasing by 26 percent.[6] There is a definite need for supplementation. However, it is becoming increasingly clear through the research that it is essential to supplement with micro- and macronutrients that are organic and come from food sources that our body recognizes.

Let us examine more closely the ways in which our food has been altered. Growing up, I remember my grandmother feeding us homemade meals with organic vegetables and fruits from her garden. The next day, I would wake up with a tremendous sense of well-being in my body. This difference was clear to me even as a child. However, many children these days are not so lucky. Due to poor farming practices like green harvesting, depleted soil, genetic modification, and widespread use of chemical fertilizers and pesticides, modern foods often lack the nutritional value they possessed just a few decades ago, and can even cause toxicity. The Department of Agriculture released a study in 2004 that illustrated a significant fall in nutrient values for forty-three vegetable products between 1950 and 1999.[7] In developed, Western countries, we often think about hunger and starvation happening "somewhere else." However, obesity, at its foundation, is often caused by an overabundance of high-caloric yet nutrient-empty foods. Just like children in developing countries, many Western children are undernourished and perpetually hungry, with deficiencies in their health at a cellular level because of a lack of healthy food. According to the World Health Organization, obesity is "one of today's most blatantly visible— yet most neglected—health problems."[8]

ANCIENT VS MODERN GRAINS

I can remember hearing commercials as a child about a popular brand of white bread. This miracle of modernity was a hybrid grain that would ensure my growth through my "formative years." I never doubted that bread, especially whole wheat bread, was good for my health, and even essential to it.

Science, however, is now understanding that altered grains—and wheat in particular— are damaging many people's intestines, immune systems, brains, and general health. Modern gluten-containing grains are proving to be less digestible and more damaging at a cellular level than glutens in grains from several decades ago. According to American neurologist Dr. David Perlmutter: "Gluten is our generation's tobacco."

Research is showing that modern gluten is the largest disrupter to our digestive health. After WWII, the food industry began altering wheat to produce higher yields using a method known as hybridization. Their intent was to feed more of the world's population more efficiently. Hybridization is when you take two different genetic strands of wheat and "breed" them through cross-pollination. There is little issue when this is done once or twice; in fact, humans have been hybridizing crops for millennia. However, these new commercial farming practices saw wheat strains "crossbred" tens of thousands of times, which altered the genetic makeup of the wheat. The visible result is that modern high-yield wheat stalks are shorter and denser than their counterparts from a century ago. The invisible result is that these new varieties of wheat contain unique glutens that are harder for most people to digest. This refined gluten has laid the foundation for an epidemic of digestive inflammation and an explosion of leaky gut syndrome.

Gluten means "glue." When ingested, it can cause the villi along the digestive tract to become shorter and inflamed. The villi in our gut should be closed and act as a barrier against what is allowed into the bloodstream and what is not. Glutens that our bodies do not recognize can eventually create small cracks or leakages in the small intestine (which covers 4,000 square feet of surface area), thereby permitting food particles to enter directly into the bloodstream. This condition is called "leaky gut syndrome." While gluten is a primary culprit in leaky gut, dairy, frequent alcohol use, pesticides, medications, and modern-day processed foods exacerbate the problem significantly. Many people suffer from leaky gut today. Many more have developed allergies, intolerances, and immune reactions to gluten, such as celiac disease. In fact, on one recent plane ride, we were asked to dispose of any and all gluten-containing products in our possession because one passenger had an extreme allergic reaction to gluten.

Understanding that modern whole wheat bread is as detrimental to our health as the nutritionally stripped white bread of my childhood was a tremendous shock for me. Growing up, and while in nursing school, I was taught that whole wheat breads and grains were better for the body because of the fiber they contained (as compared to more processed white breads and grains). Realizing that modern wheat bread has a higher glycemic index than a candy bar and as such is a huge contributor to the obesity and diabetes epidemics floored me. Furthermore, learning that modern wheat has been so altered that our bodies do not recognize its glutens anymore, I found myself asking, "What grains can I eat that won't hurt me?"

At a lecture by Larry Law, I was surprised to learn that there are ancient grains and seeds still available to consumers. With these heirloom flours and seeds, I can bake bread, eat pasta, and even make healthier cakes! These ancient grains are einkorn, emmer, kamut, amaranth, quinoa, millet, sorghum, chia, teff, freekeh, buckwheat, and spelt (although spelt does contain some gluten). Of course, anything rice-based will also be gluten free (although checking the ingredients list is always advisable).

The foundation of creating and sustaining a healthy body is to nourish it with good, high-frequency primary and secondary foods. Yet, how can we live optimally when the majority of our food does not sustain cell health? The consequence of our current food production methods is that many, if not most, of us are starving at a cellular level. We are craving the nutrients that are missing and, as a result, overeating foods that are high in calories and processed sugar but low in nutrients.

Our food industry has been operating from a lack of integrity for decades, and it no longer serves humanity at this time. We need a new system to provide and support us in getting the foods that truly nourish us. Despite this "nutritional illusion" at play in our food and healthcare markets, all is not lost. We can still try to choose whole, organic, locally produced foods when possible, and supplement them with organic freeze-dried vitamins and minerals. Simple choices like these will tremendously influence the health and vitality of our bodies.

Food, the Gut, and our Immune System

As science is showing the strong connection between the health of our gut and the health of our immune system, we are understanding on a much deeper level that food truly matters. Some say that the health of our gut determines the health of our whole body.

Our immune system is our body's innate sensory protection system. It was created to protect the body, mind, and spirit from anything that could cause imbalances, injuries, or attacks. Our skin is our first line of defense against outside invaders, and our digestive system is our "second skin." Lymph nodes line the intestines, regulating and modulating what is needed and allowed to remain in the body, and what is not. The intelligence of the lymph system is on high alert for toxins and invaders. On a spiritual level, there is a connection between the boundaries we place in our life and the physical boundaries the complex gut immune system places. As we learn to make decisions about what is good for us and what is not, we are mirroring what our gut should do for us every hour of every day. If you think of your immune system as a "boundary enforcer," you will more clearly understand its function.

In previous chapters, we looked at how we have thus far lived life through a dualistic lens. Everything we do, our cells mirror. The roles of victim, perpetrator, and savior have been played out at the cellular level as well. A potential victim could be represented by our vulnerability at the cell level by anything that may attack/harm us. The perpetrator role could be represented by the harmful bacteria, parasites, viruses, and fungi. Parasites exist on all levels of body, mind, and spirit. People can be "parasitic" when they are unable to own their own Creatorship and need to drain and pull energy from others. On the other hand, high-frequency bacteria, viruses, and fungi often play the role of the savior as they are constantly rebalancing and upgrading the system.

In this section, we'll look at the microbiome, which is the ecosystem of bacteria, viruses, fungi, and cells that make up the human body. While the microbiome is part of all of our organs and systems, when speaking about it we usually focus on three areas: the gut, the skin, and the brain. A healthy microbiome has been scientifically shown to prevent many of the imbalances or illnesses that we see today, including inflammatory bowel diseases, obesity, brain disorders, cancer, and asthma allergies, to name a few. The microbiome also helps us to eliminate toxins and helps us create necessary boundaries along our digestive tract for protective purposes.

Now, let's look at bacteria.

Did you know that we have more bacteria in our bodies than we do cells? In fact, we have around ten bacteria for every single human cell. There are smaller numbers of bacteria in the stomach and small intestines; the majority of our bacterial microbiome can be found in the large intestine.

From the origin of our species, the survival of humanity has depended on our ability to exchange genetic information. This has also been the case for bacteria. Bacteria need nutrition much like we do. They need sources of carbon, nitrogen, sulfur, phosphorus, and minerals. At this time, the bacteria in our microbiome get their energy from carbon-based sources like sugars, proteins, amino acids, and fats. They can also get energy from the transfer of electrons and can use photosynthesis to get their light energy from adenosine triphosphate (ATP), the energy-carrying molecule found in cells.[9]

Why are bacteria so important to our health and well-being? Because they are part of us! They cover the entire body (skin); all orifices including the mouth, vagina, and rectum; and the large intestine of our digestive tract. They also play the largest role in our gut health. The primary role of bacteria in the gut is to help us digest our food and absorb nutrients. Our intestines decide what gets passed into the body and brain from our food. There is a strong connection between the gut and the brain; they even resemble each other physically.

I learned this the hard way. While traveling, I would often become sick as a result of exposure to unfamiliar bacteria and new foods. After suffering with giardia for a year, I noticed I began to become very anxious, overwhelmed, and have panic attacks. I thought it was from the stress in my life. Although that was certainly part of it, I wish I had known then what I know today: namely, that gut bacteria are responsible for making the neurotransmitters (serotonin, dopamine) that our brain needs for optimal function. In order to conduct a thought, the brain must send an impulse of information over a synapse. When there are enough neurotransmitters, our mood and ability to focus are optimal. However, if there are not enough neurotransmitters, the brain slows down, and messages cannot be sent properly. In this way, the bacteria in our gut are partially responsible for our brain health.

The quality of our food and the medicines we take directly influence our microbiome health. If we only eat processed foods, we run the risk of cultivating fewer strains of good bacteria, which can create an unhealthy microbiome. Antibiotics (which are, in my opinion, over-prescribed throughout the world) can wipe out good bacteria in the gut as well as the invaders that are making us sick. Research published by The Human Microbiome Project reported that the microbiome, which had previously been assumed to include 700 species of bacteria, in fact contained closer to 10,000 different types, and most of them were contained within the large intestine. It was also noted that the number and diversity of species of bacteria determines the health of the intestines. When the "good" (higher frequency) bacteria outnumber the "bad" (lower frequency) bacteria, the health of the gut is kept in balance. When the bad bacteria start to overpower the good, imbalances start to happen throughout the gut and brain.[10] Knowing this, I now better understand the consequences of having taken so many antibiotics to get rid of the giardia!

We receive our microbiome at birth. As the water breaks and the baby comes through the vaginal canal, the baby is bathed in the bacteria from the mother's vagina and rectum. As I have already mentioned, my eldest son was born by cesarean section and therefore did not receive this inoculation of healthy bacteria; I believe that this contributed to his immune struggles in his first few years of life.

Later in life, we continue to grow our microbiome every time we eat fresh food and are outside in nature. Where we live will affect our unique flora. When the microbiome lacks diversity due to these factors and others, it becomes imbalanced and vulnerable to pathogens, antibiotic-resistant bacteria, and invaders, as our boundaries are down.

In Dr. Perlmutter's book *Grain Brain: The Surprising Truth about Wheat, Carbs, and Sugar—Your Brain's Silent Killers*, he teaches that foods high in altered grains cause inflammation both in the gut as well as the brain. Chronic inflammation is one of the largest obstacles to a healthy functioning gut, brain, and immune system. The word "inflammation" comes from the Latin word *inflammare*, "to ignite." Having inflammation in the body blocks cell-to-cell communication, the transport system in the body, nutrient absorption and distribution, and the clean-up system, among others.

Like all other aspects of our being, immune healing takes place at all levels. Stress, eating unhealthy foods, too many low-frequency emotions, too little or too much activity, drinking alcohol to excess, smoking, and other lifestyle choices can all contribute to inflammation.

When I began to focus on improving my immune system, I started with my emotions and stress. As I learned to meditate and worked with José to release blocked emotions and genetic baggage, I also became more interested in changing the foods I was eating. These days, eating anti-inflammatory foods is a routine for me. I love drinking smoothies in the summer with organic kale, celery, apples, spinach, avocado, ginger, blueberries, raspberries, or blackberries. I also try to eat more fresh fruits and green salads during the summer months. In the colder months, I try to incorporate warming vegetable soups or plain vegetables with every meal. If I feel like having fruits in the winter, I often warm them up; I also steam my vegetables or bake them with some olive oil. My favorites are cauliflower, asparagus, cabbage, endives, pumpkin, sea vegetables, tomatoes, zucchini, and onions. It took time for me to change old habits of eating too many animal proteins and processed foods, but now I truly enjoy and appreciate my more natural diet.

Food is Information: Restoring Our Frequency

As we discussed in Chapter Six, everything is made up of energy, and everything has a frequency. Foods are also made of energy, and each has a unique frequency. In fact, food is information. Just like hormones carry different messages, food also carries different messages, and (as we learned above) can impact the epigenome. Since you become what you eat, the frequency of your food will influence the frequency of your Creator Matrix on all levels. As you grow in consciousness, all aspects of your Creator Matrix as a unit will vibrate higher and higher. In other words, your Creator Matrix will be holding a frequency that will itself influence which foods you choose, and which foods serve your system. As your Creator Matrix becomes more integrated, so too will your ability to shift your frequency, and then perhaps even low-frequency foods could have a less damaging impact on you. Your beliefs can and will influence how food (and anything) can influence you. The consciousness of how you interact with food will determine how food affects you and how you choose your food.

Some foods naturally have a higher frequency and hold more light for rejuvenation. The highest-frequency foods include, but are not limited to, green leafy vegetables, fresh berries, microgreens and sprouts, herbs, legumes, and nuts. On the other hand, other foods have lower frequencies and hold less light. In fact, some "foods" (including many processed foods) have no life force at all, thereby prompting the body to recognize them as toxins rather than sources of nutrition and high-frequency information. Again, as mentioned in Chapter Six, when we become sick, our body is at a lower frequency. It is then up to us and the body to heal by raising our frequency. One way to do this is by consciously focusing on positive thoughts and emotions. Another way is by eating high-frequency foods that have ample life force. According to the Institute of Transformational Nutrition:

- Healthy body frequency: 62–72 MHz
- Fresh foods: 20–27 MHz (higher if grown organically)
- Dried foods: 15–22 MHz
- Processed foods: 0 MHz[11]

Kirlian photography (which we touched on briefly in Chapter Six) was developed in 1939 and creates photos with an electrified photographic plate. Many people believe that these photographs represent the auras, biofield, or energy of chi that surrounds objects, plants, animals, and people. Natural foods, nurtured and cared for, contain light that is restorative to our health and well-being. When foods vibrate at a higher frequency, they contain more light.

Below are three images of foods and the light they emit. These photos by Nigel Hutchings of Fullspectrum.org.uk provide powerful confirmation of how important it is to be conscious of the foods we eat daily. Food not only builds our cells and gives us energy, but also (and more significantly) restores our light and raises our frequency.

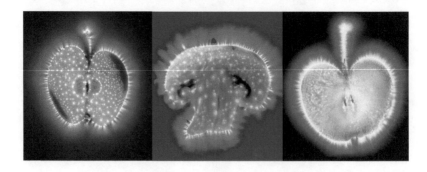

Our thoughts about food are just as important as the food itself. As we grow in consciousness, all areas of our life will change; this includes our relationship with food. Connecting with food and choosing our own frequency means making food choices that are healthier and that suit our bio-individuality. Consciously connecting to the foods we choose is a very important part of the process. Staying present with food as we eat it can have a powerful effect on how it interacts with our system. When we enjoy the food and allow ourselves to experience feelings of joy as we eat it, we influence the way our body interacts with the food. If we feel low-frequency emotions while eating due to unresolved feelings throughout our body, this will affect the way the food interacts with us at the cellular level.

I remember going to a clinic for a detox program. To my surprise, I was given a very small portion of food for each meal. During the week, I became accustomed to eating my food very slowly and savoring each small bite. By the end of the week, my entire consciousness and relationship with food had changed. I was not just filling an empty void; I was becoming one with the food as I ate it, and it was becoming one with me.

Our collective belief systems around food and nourishment are also important. We need to look closely at what we've created and assess whether our inherited or learned beliefs still hold true, and whether the systems we've created are still serving us around food, farming, and distribution. Take, for example, the differences between commercial and organic farming. Commercial farming was born from the desire to feed more people quickly, and did not respect the laws of nature. It did not take into account the negative effects of commercial toxic pesticides on the soil and plants as well as people. It neglected the importance of the diversity of soil microbes for health. On the other hand, organic farming respects the need to rotate crops, respects the need for soil to be diverse and rest, and uses natural methods to control unwanted pests. There are also important frequency differences between grain-fed and grass-fed beef, and between caged chickens who never see daylight and free-roaming chickens eating their natural diet instead of grains; in both cases, the free-range options are more nutritious. Unfortunately, organic meats and vegetables cost more to produce, making them unaffordable for many. However, the more people become aware of how their food is serving them, the more demand there will be for higher-quality products. Ultimately, our collective choices can and will alter market conditions.

Processed foods carry their own energies, too. Sugary pastries, cereals, and drinks taste good, but they're made in factories. Little love and care go into their preparation. Moreover, they are threatening the health of millions on a daily basis due to their lack of nutrition and information. They directly contribute to the global epidemics of diabetes and obesity. When we become cognizant of the damage certain foods are doing collectively, they may become less appealing to us individually.

Next time you go to the market, observe how you feel about certain foods or food products. As you grow in consciousness, you will begin to receive intuitive information about what does and does not serve your body at this time.

Weight Management and Neuroscience

It is not always easy to live in our dualistic world. For some, it's unbearable.

Personally, my journey into expanded consciousness has given me tremendous love and admiration for us as humans. Again, I think we are all heroes for being willing to come to Earth and live as physical beings during such chaotic times. With all the violence, conflict, and uncertainty happening now, many of us feel very unsafe. The root cause of aggression is often fear—which, as we know, is a frequency that does not serve our body, mind, or spirit at all.

Our uncertainty, fear, and negativity have been mirrored in our relationship with food. And at the same time, we become what we eat. We also "become" as we integrate our life experiences and allow them to change and evolve us. As the Creator in our life, we are in a constant state of transforming and becoming. With the sudden rise of consciousness, this process has been accelerating. Many people find it difficult to make all these changes alongside conducting a human life here on Earth. This is reflected in the global issues we are having around food and our weight management.

Our physical bodies are always affected by what we are feeling, and they let us know how we are doing. We looked at how stress affects our bodies and can contribute to weight gain in Chapter Four. When we feel exhausted with life and our life force is low, it can be very hard to take in life force through food. As a result, we can undernourish ourselves or develop habits of overeating (taking in too much). Many eating disorders have an emotional/spiritual component as well.

Although each person has their own relationship to food, there are some basic issues that show up again and again for my clients who are working on weight management issues. Food brings us something on all levels! At the physical, cellular level the macronutrient of fat protects our cells and gives them support. Fat also helps our bodies (and us) to feel safe and protected. As mentioned earlier, food helps us emotionally digest our life stories, process what we need from them, and let go of what we don't need. On a spiritual level, food helps us to be here on Earth—to ground, connect to ourselves and others, nourish our spirit, bring comfort, safety, and protection. When we have not learned how to do this, we can suffer from imbalances with food intake. Food helps life to feel more palatable for us. Having too little or too much fat around our cells and in our bodies can be a sign of feeling unsafe and vulnerable, and also reflect a lack of self-worth and self-love.

An Ayurvedic doctor I'm acquainted with once asked his client, "What is the food bringing you?"

The client answered, "Sweetness."

The doctor replied, "In what areas of your life have you not been receiving sweetness?"

She immediately started crying. "My husband has no time to talk to me and is often unkind."

The doctor continued, "How is the food serving you?"

She answered, "It helps me feel better and brings me comfort."

As I listened to this story, I immediately thought about an infant crying with feelings of hunger and abandonment. I could imagine the relief felt by the infant once the mother gave her milk—and the safety it represented—again and again.

As Creators, we must learn to create safety here on Earth for ourselves. Once I understood this, I understood that food-related imbalances do serve us in some ways.

Obesity has become a global epidemic. Obesity-related diseases are among the top three killers in most developed countries. We live in an obesogenic environment, meaning that our society contributes to many factors that support people in becoming obese. On a physical level, as we explored earlier, the foods that we are eating are stimulating food addictions. Eating too much food with little nutrition can lead to malnutrition, regardless of a person's current weight. Processed foods with too few nutrients and too little life force energy leave people unsatisfied at the cellular level. When this happens, the body continues to signal the need to eat as the cells are searching for the nutrition they need to function.

Neuroscientists have examined how processed, low-nutrient foods affect our brain and habits. The chemical substances in these foods produce feelings of euphoria which help people feel better immediately and therefore cope with their current stressors, fears, and anxieties. When you eat something that tastes good, particularly something high in sugar, you stimulate the dopamine reward pathway, just as you would by having sex or taking drugs like cocaine. When this area of the brain is stimulated, increasing amounts of dopamine are released. However, as this pathway becomes overstimulated, the system becomes out of balance and the body signals for more stimulants. Studies in rats have found that Oreo cookies were as addictive as drugs like cocaine to test subjects, and that the high fat/high sugar content stimulated the pleasure reward center of the brain in the same way as hard drugs do.[12]

Many hormones besides dopamine are released in relation to what we eat, including leptin and ghrelin. Leptin signals to the system that we are satisfied (and therefore should stop eating), while ghrelin signals that we are unsatisfied and need to eat. Those who are overweight tend to have plenty of leptin, however the use of it can become blocked. How does this happen? As we eat more and more refined sugar and processed foods like pastries, pasta, bread, and soda, the pancreas must work very hard to manage the high level of sugar in the body. Insulin docks on cell receptors to allow the sugar into the cell for use. After a while, the cells which have been fed enough sugar obstruct the insulin from bringing more sugar; this is called insulin resistance, and it is considered a precursor to diabetes. When this happens, the pancreas becomes depleted and is unable to keep releasing insulin. One can of cola contains nearly ten teaspoons of sugar. Imagine what just one can a day can do to your pancreas! But let's get back to the problem with leptin. Leptin is released according to the amount of fat on your body. The more fat you have, the higher your leptin levels will be. However, if you keep feeding your body more than it needs, your cells will block the leptin and you will get leptin resistance. When leptin receptors are blocked, the message that you are full is also blocked, so ghrelin takes over, signaling that you are still hungry. It is a vicious cycle. Crash diets only make things worse. Leptin is trying to help maintain weight in the long term. When you lose weight suddenly, your body fat decreases, and so do your leptin levels. This can signal your body to think you are starving, which of course stimulates you to eat more. This is a key reason why many people cannot stick with restrictive or low-calorie diets in the long term.

So, what are the solutions? A holistic approach is often best. Managing stress more effectively, reprogramming limited beliefs about food and emotions, becoming more conscious of our relationship with food through trial and error, and working to find the best variety of foods that nourish us can all support weight loss. Artificial intelligence will also offer solutions. There are machines on the market that can tell us what foods can nourish us the best from day to day. I believe each person must find their own way and that there is no "one size fits all" approach.

I myself have struggled with being overweight after menopause.

The only solution that worked was realizing that my eating behaviors had to change permanently in this stage of life. This required a change in both my lifestyle and my relationship to food. I first had to recognize that I was addicted to sugar and get off it completely. Then, I had to find foods that served me. I also found a health coach, Lia, and an emotional healer to help me through this process. The emotional healer offered me an outlet to reprogram my limiting beliefs about worthiness, and my Lia offered me support and accountability as I cut out the sugar and starches that were constantly sabotaging my progress. I had to become more organized in my daily food intake. I also had to find what worked best for me, which ended up being foods that stimulated ketosis and put my system into "fat-burning" mode. This helped me to control my sugar cravings. Together, Lia and I were able to come up with strategies for what to eat when I had cravings. She also guided me to find exercises that I liked and could continue to fit in my busy schedule. And, while there are "quick fix" solutions on the market—like new drugs and surgeries—I knew these were not for me and would not support me in the long term. If I truly wanted to heal at all levels of my body, mind, spirit matrix, I needed to learn to love and accept myself as I am, not alter my body to fit someone else's idea of "health."

If you are also struggling with excess weight or any imbalance around food, I suggest you start with love and acceptance for all aspects of yourself, including your body. As Creators, we can change our reality once we truly step into our authentic power. Refusing to accept and love ourselves will make it much harder to become the Creators we are meant to be.

We Are What We Eat

Knowing that we are what we eat is essential. Food is vitally important for the health of our body, mind, and spirit matrix. When we wake up each morning feeling fatigued, grumpy, and with little life force, we cannot do what we are here on Earth to do. Feeling less than optimal is not serving us.

Humanity must take a step forward to clean up our food, environment, and water systems. We need to clean up Mother Earth! As Creators, we need to collectively take and demand action. The future of our health and wellness, and the futures of our children, depends upon it.

In the next chapter, we will dive into the new science of glycobiology and look further at how our primary and secondary foods affect our cellular wellness.

Chapter Summary

- When we grow in consciousness, we begin to observe the food choices we make and our habits around eating. Making changes in this area is often the first step toward becoming more conscious of all areas in our life.

- Nutrigenomics looks at the effect of food on gene expression, while nutrigenetics looks at how people's genetics influence the ways in which their body will react or respond to certain foods. In this way, food is information.

- Gut issues have an emotional aspect and a physical component.

- Food choices can change gene expression. What we eat matters because food is information. We live on a toxic planet. Making conscious lifestyle choices matters.

- The food we eat is more than just fuel for energy. We become what we eat: the million cells per second that we make need the right building blocks from the food we eat in order to create proper functioning structures.

- Nutrient values of our foods have declined significantly due to less-healthy farming practices like green harvesting, soil depletion, genetic modification, and widespread use of chemical fertilizers and pesticides.

- Modern altered (hybridized) gluten-containing grains are less digestible and more damaging at a cellular level than ancient grains, causing inflammation in the gut and brain, leaky gut, and the epidemic of diabetes and obesity.

- The microbiome—the community of microorganisms in the human body—plays the largest role in our gut health, helping us to create boundaries along the digestive tract and eliminating toxins. Bacteria in the gut help us digest our food, absorb nutrients, and make neurotransmitters (serotonin, dopamine) that our brain needs for optimal function.

- Chronic inflammation is one of the largest obstacles to a healthy functioning gut, brain, and immune system. It blocks cell-to-cell communication, the transport system in the body, nutrient absorption and distribution, and the clean-up system.

- Foods have energy and a frequency. Eating high-frequency foods with life force is important to rejuvenate our bodies and restore our frequency.

- As we grow in consciousness, we will begin to receive intuitive information about what food does and does not serve our body at this time. Until then, we can choose whole, organic, locally produced foods, grass-fed organic beef, and organic free-range eggs supplemented with natural freeze-dried vitamins and minerals.

Chapter Nine

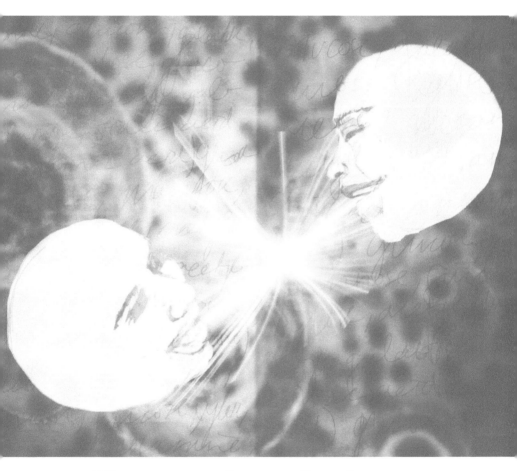

*How can understanding how our
cells connect help us understand
our health and well-being?*

"Everything you'll ever need to know is within you; the secrets of the universe are imprinted on the cells of your body."

- Dan Millman

CHAPTER NINE

Glycoscience

E veryone can relate to the idea and feeling of being lost. This concept can apply at all levels of existence. On a physical level, we can actually become lost and find ourselves in unfamiliar surroundings. Imagine a young child realizing that they've lost their parents at the local fair or shopping mall; this experience can leave them feeling panicked, fearful, and disorientated. Likewise, on a mental or spiritual level, we often hear people say, "I feel lost," or, "I'm not sure how to go forward." This experience can create similar levels of uncertainty and fear.

In all my years helping people heal, I have realized that healing has little to do with "fixing" what is not working, and everything to do with reconnecting on all levels of the body, mind, and spirit matrix. To heal is to become whole—to reconnect and find oneself again. This self-re-unification can lead to feelings of clarity, cohesiveness, and empowerment, and guide us toward a renewed sense of purpose and direction.

Thus far in this book, we have been discussing the principles of connection and disconnection on all levels of existence: physical, mental, and spiritual. Our cells also exist on all these levels. When our cells are disconnected, they can become disorientated and chaotic. In essence, they are "lost," unable to navigate themselves through their environment and disconnected from their purpose. We are constantly influencing our cells, and our cells are influencing us. We can't find health without understanding how important cellular connection and communication is.

When I moved to the Netherlands, I attended many conferences concerning the mind, body, spirit, and healing connection. One day, while reading, I came across a concept that struck me. The author of this research asserted that cells communicate with one another, and that poor cell communication was a major cause of imbalance and disease in the body. This brought to mind the many patients I'd met over the years who seemed disconnected from their bodies and had no idea why they had become ill. Looking back, many of them also seemed disconnected from their essence and their emotions, as well as their physical state. Could this disconnection be mirrored in our cells? Could a lack of cell connection and diminished cell-to-cell communication be responsible for a lack of body-to-mind communication?

Several weeks later, I received a tragic phone call. My cousin had been shot and killed, and the family was in shock. Within a week, I flew back to the US to attend his funeral in Chicago. At the funeral, another cousin approached me, and asked, "Cathleen, have you ever heard of glycoscience? Did you know that your cells communicate constantly, every second of every day?" Synchronicity is an interesting thing. To be honest, I was not very open to the conversation at that moment since I was busy trying to console family members and digest my own grief. Still, I wondered why this information was showing up again. My cousin continued. "Our bodies make millions of new cells every second, and how those cells are made matters." At that moment, the conversation no longer felt inconvenient. It felt like a door had just opened to my new path of study—and now that it was open, I could not ignore it. The big question I had was, "If this science is so vital to our health and wellness, why haven't I heard about it? Why hasn't anyone I know heard about it?" From that moment on, I was driven to understand the importance of cell-to-cell communication and its significance to the wellness of our whole being.

Cell-to-cell communication comprises the "telephone" network through which our cells "speak" to one another. This science is called glycoscience.

What is Glycoscience?

Glycoscience is the study of glycans (also known as sugar chains) and how they function in the body. These are not the sugars we know as food ingredients—which are usually sweet, refined, and full of empty calories—but rather a group of eight specific carbohydrates that form a type of "cellular alphabet" that is the basis for all cell-to-cell communication. These eight sugars are glucose, galactose, mannose, fucose, xylose, acetyl glucosamine, acetyl galactosamine, and sialic acid (neuraminic acid). They exist everywhere in nature and are around every cell in every living organism. They should be found in many of our fruits and vegetables, however, as mentioned earlier, many nutrients have been removed from our food due to modern agricultural methods and food processing, and this includes glycans. There are over 200 carbohydrates in nature and only eight of them (glycans) are responsible for cell communication. They look like a forest on the cell surface.

Glycans are arranged in many different combinations, and there seems to be a universal electromagnetic field of energy that helps glycans transmit information. This is a multidimensional process that can be influenced by all fields of existence: physical, mental, emotional, and spiritual. This has made it difficult for scientists and tech companies to understand all the possible combinations that cells can make to communicate. While protein structures in DNA are structured linearly, like wagon trains, glycans are multidimensional; like the branches on a tree, they can go in all directions. Glycans are made in structures that combine with other macromolecules in the body (proteins and fats) to carry out cell functions. When glycans are connected to proteins, they are called glycoproteins; when they are connected to fats, they are called glycolipids. Together the glycoproteins and glycolipids are referred to as glycoconjugates. The glycoproteins in the cell membrane accept the signal, decipher it, and process it into the cell. This glycoprotein changes shape depending on the message and how it interacts with the molecules around it.

CELL MEMBRANE

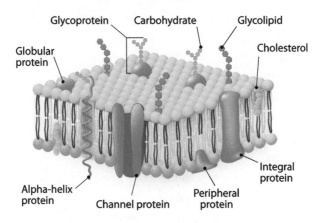

THE GEOMETRY OF THE BODY: GLYCANS AND CELL FUNCTION

In 2012, the National Academy of Science (NAS) outlined a roadmap on how to bring the knowledge of glycoscience to the masses and increase the research being done on it. However, they also pointed out hurdles to research pathways, saying, "Glycans have received little attention from the research community due, in large part, to a lack of tools to probe their often-complex structures and properties."[1]

When I read the NAS report, I was struck by several powerful conclusions that were made in its text. The first was, "Glycans play roles in almost every biological process and are involved in every major disease."

That statement got my attention. Glycans are obviously very important and are involved in almost every biological process and disease state.

The second concept that struck me was that glycans determine the differences in human blood groups. The sugars on the cell membrane are referred to as the glycocalyx. The glycocalyx of the red blood cells form the basis of the four different blood groups (A, B, AB & O). Each blood group has the same red blood cell but a different terminal (last) sugar (glycan) on the sugar strands/antennas on the cell surface; this determines its unique blood group. As a nurse, I know that knowing somebody's blood type can mean the difference between life or death. When we had to give people blood transfusions in the hospital, it was vitally important that we double-checked a person's blood group. If we gave a patient blood of the wrong type, there would be an instant breakdown in cell communication because of the difference in glycan codes. In essence, the immune system would fail to recognize the terminal sugar as "self," so it would see the donated blood cells as foreign invaders and work to destroy them. This reaction would cause cellular breakdown, which can lead to death.

Finally, the NAS further stated that, "Elimination of any single major class of glycans from an organism results in death." This information is significant as it strongly reinforces how important the cell membrane is; as I mentioned earlier, the cell membrane, not the nucleus, is the command center or "brain" of the cell. As we learned in Chapter Seven, the cell nucleus is much like a library; it stores information in the DNA that offers us many potentialities and possibilities that can be expressed, manifested, and experienced. When we enter a library, we can choose any book on any shelf to read; we do not have to read every single book in the library, nor do all books need to be read for the library to continue existing. A cell can live for months if the nucleus is removed—however, if we take just one class of sugars off the cell membrane, the cell will die immediately. In other words, glycans are crucial to the fate and health of any cell; the body cares about these sugars, and we are only beginning to understand how much.

In this way, glycoscience is radically changing our understanding of the human cell and how it functions at all levels—and, therefore, how we function as whole beings.

Realizing how important the structures of the membranes are, I now understood that the body cares about how cells are built, and also how cellular structures are put together. The body relies on perfect geometry. It maintains the architecture of the molecules that control the function. Again, structure is function. If the cell membrane is pivotal to the behavior and fate of the cell, the next question must then be, "Who or what is in charge of the membrane?" On a holistic or multidimensional level, we as Creators are in control. However, at the cellular level, glycans—or, more accurately, glycoconjugate struc-tures—are running the show.

Along my path, I met a group of glycobiologists who are part of a company called Glycan Age. They are researching the age of people's cells by looking at the structure and combinations of glycans on the outside of every cell (glycocalyx) through blood analysis. They analyze the different glycan combinations, and based on which glycans are there and which are absent, they are able to determine a person's true biolog-ical age. Their research clearly shows that a person's lifestyle choices—including food intake, traumas, and emotional health—tremendously impact the health and true biological age of one's cells.[2] There is much that we don't yet know, but one thing is abundantly clear: glycans are just as powerful as our DNA!

As Creators, we have learned that our thoughts and emotions send signals of information that influence our environment, our well-being, and ultimately our reality. The body has its own network of intelligence and communicates messages through cell signaling. Communication from our consciousness, mind, and emotions are transmitted clearly with the support of glycans. Glycans act like antennas that are responsi-ble for our cells' ability to communicate. Messages are sent every second in real time at the cell level based on the needs of the body, mind, and spirit. These antennas cover all the cells in our body, and work by picking up the frequencies of tiny particles inside atoms that are wiggling back and forth (vibrating) with an ability to receive and send signals of information. At the cell membrane, the glycans are checking and connecting with anything that wants to engage with the cell.

Every one of us has our own unique code surrounding our cells that ensures cell self-recognition. The glycans surrounding each cell are constantly checking everything in their environment to make sure they have the correct "self-code." When something in the body does not possess this self-code, the immune system is instructed to destroy the invader. Signals received by the cell membrane are then transmitted into the cell, where they influence what structures will be made to carry out the needed cell activities. The process by which signals are sent from the membrane into the cell is known as signal transduction. Other signals are sent to the nucleus to pull up data from the DNA in order to instruct the ribosomes to make needed protein structures.

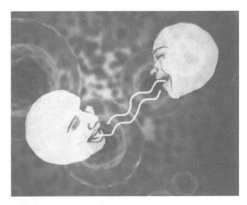

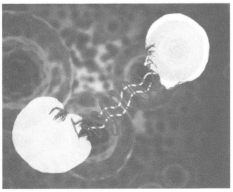

When cell communication is clear, cells can function easily and coherently; however, when cell communication is not clear, cells are unable to function optimally. If our cell communication is impaired at any level, we cannot be truly healthy.

The Missing Link in Nutrition

As my research continued, it became increasingly clear that there was a difference between glycoscience (glycobiology) and nutritional glycoscience. In the former, researchers are more focused on glycans in terms of disease process and pharmacology. In nutritional glycoscience, however, the focus is on the glycans' relationship to food and nourishment.

Both aspects of glycoscience are being studied at top universities. In fact, the 2003 MIT Technology Review publication, *Glycomics,* listed glycoscience as one of the "Top 10 Emerging Technologies that Will Change the World." But, if this is true, why is the research on glycoscience talked about so little, even in medical circles?

Doctors and nurses are not generally given much instruction on nutrition. They are under tremendous pressure and stress and are often unaware and/or unable to care for themselves and eat properly during their long shifts. During my own nursing training, nutritional science was not even part of the curriculum. As my research continued, I realized that nutrition could provide the basis for understanding how our cells should function optimally. Nutritional science looks at the interaction between the substances in food (nutrients) that contribute to a cell's ability to grow, repair, and maintain health. As I discovered more about glycoscience, I realized that it provided the missing piece to the puzzle of nutritional science. I decided, therefore, to incorporate more of these glycans into my diet. Not only did I notice an improvement in my overall health, but I also felt a stronger spiritual connection to my higher self and to Mother Earth. It felt as if my circuitry was back online.

Let's look exactly at how glycans are utilized by the body through food. Our food is made up of macromolecules (macronutrients): proteins, fats, and carbohydrates (including glycans). We become what we eat; macronutrients make up all the building blocks of our cells, therefore the macronutrients we consume become the structure of new cells. How does this happen? When food is eaten, the body begins to break down the macronutrients for absorption. The proteins are broken down into amino acids, fats into fatty acids, and carbohydrates into monosaccharides including the eight glycans. Many of these nutrients are taken into the cell via the cell membrane through a process called endocytosis. Once in the cell, these structures are sent to the endoplasmic reticulum or the golgi apparatus for restructuring and packaging based on the needs of the cell at a particular moment. When sugars are added to proteins or lipids, the process is called glycosylation. This biochemical process is ongoing. If glycans are the means by which our cells perceive and share information, it becomes essential that the glycan structure is well made so it can transmit accurate messages.

It is important to understand that we need to access glycans through our diet to build healthy cells. Since the food we eat is compromised and largely deficient in necessary nutrients, this lack of glycans will eventually cause problems with proper glycosylation and cell communication. When communication is clear, the body can function optimally. However, when communication is hampered in any way, chaos can result, which can lead to altered or aberrant glycosylation. It is a vicious cycle.

As Drs. Alavi and Axford noted in their 2008 report, "Sweet and Sour: The Impact of Sugar on Disease": "Aberrant changes in cellular processes, such as those that accompany disease, are therefore likely to result in alterations of the glycan profiles of the cell surface and/or secreted glycoconjugates, in particular glycoproteins. And so, not surprisingly, most major diseases, when probed, are found to be directly/indirectly associated with a change in the glycosylation pattern of at least one central structure."[3]

After learning about the importance of glycans for cell communication, I continued to search for answers to what causes the alterations in the glycan profile that are contributing to so many diseases on the planet. Diseases like cancer are not only caused by something, but by the *lack* of something. Here I was brought back again to the tremendous power nutrition plays in our health and wellness and the detrimental effects caused by the lack of it, especially a lack of glycans. Scientist Larry Law, in addressing the pathogenesis of cancer, states, "When glycosylation goes awry, sugars are not where they should be, and cancer can result and progress."[4] This implies that missing sugars are impacting our nourishment, and therefore our cellular health, connection, and communication.

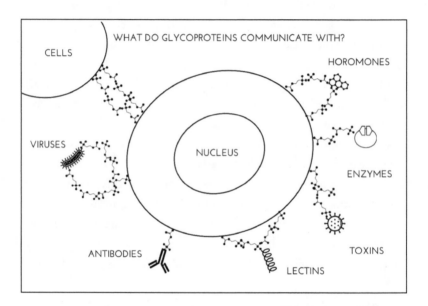

WHAT DO GLYCOPROTEINS COMMUNICATE WITH?

CELLS

HOROMONES

VIRUSES

NUCLEUS

ENZYMES

ANTIBODIES

TOXINS

LECTINS

I began to wonder exactly what glycans were connecting and communicating with at the level of the cell membrane. It turns out that glycans communicate with *everything* in their environment—all of the nutrients (lectins), hormones, enzymes, viruses, bacteria, toxins, antibodies, other microorganisms, and anything else that interacts with the cell.[5][6]

As I was teaching about this new science, I came up with a few metaphors that helped my students to understand the power of glycans. I compare glycans to "guardians" who act as cells' doormen, determining what the cell will allow in and what it will keep out based on the

needs of the cell in real time. I have also compared glycans to the conductor of an orchestra. As the conductor oversees the timing and connections between each instrument and each part of the symphony, so
too do glycans oversee all communications and interactions within and
between our cells. If an orchestra is missing its conductor, the music will
be affected and may become chaotic; without glycans "conducting" the
normal activities of the cell, those activities can be affected. Messages
between cells can become scrambled and confused, which can lead to
miscommunication within the body.

Since glycans are used by the body to send signals both within and
between cells, without them the cells are unable to support and sustain
even the simple everyday tasks that sustain life. Just as we must nourish
ourselves daily, eliminate toxins, protect ourselves from hazards, and
connect with our world in order to thrive, so too must our cells! We
and our cells are connected.

Perhaps research in the future will study all aspects of our body-
mind-spirit Creator Matrix in a more holistic way. Focusing on our
new understanding of glycoscience can help us to find more optimal
wellness at the cellular level. When our cells are communicating well,
we can be on our journey to manifesting optimal wellness.

CELL SIGNALING CONTROLS ACTIVITIES
THAT MAINTAIN HEALTH

My new passion for understanding glycoscience was fueled by the
vast numbers of people who are suffering from diseases and/or simply
having trouble performing the daily activities of life. I wanted to understand what exactly glycans do to maintain the health of our cells. To
understand this better, I needed to focus on what cells do in general.

Cells need to perform certain tasks daily to stay healthy, much like we
do. They eat, drink, breathe, and release toxins on a daily basis. Imagine
that a cell needs certain nutrients; however, because of poor communication, it cannot identify the nutrients it needs. Or, suppose the cell has
become very toxic; however, due to poor cell communication, the cell has

trouble identifying and releasing the toxins.

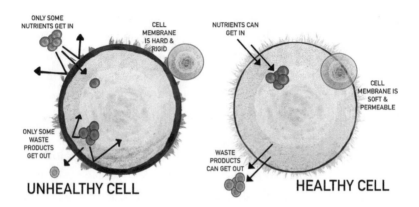

ONLY SOME NUTRIENTS GET IN

CELL MEMBRANE IS HARD & RIGID

ONLY SOME WASTE PRODUCTS GET OUT

UNHEALTHY CELL

NUTRIENTS CAN GET IN

CELL MEMBRANE IS SOFT & PERMEABLE

WASTE PRODUCTS CAN GET OUT

HEALTHY CELL

Imagine that someone is hemorrhaging after an accident, and the cells are sending messages to stop the bleeding. However, due to poor cell communication, the messages are being misunderstood. Consequently, the body's reaction to stop the bleeding is too slow, and the person requires a transfusion—or even bleeds to death. Or imagine that someone ate food contaminated with bacteria, but because of poor cell communication in their gut, the cells cannot identify the invader. The immune system, therefore, is slow to respond, resulting in weeks or months of sickness for the person.

Glycans are involved in every biological process supporting life. Here is a small list of the roles glycans play in cellular activities in our bodies: cellular respiration (cells convert sugars into energy); cellular eating (phagocytosis); cellular drinking (pinocytosis); removing toxins and wastes (exocytosis); cellular protection (immunity); making cell structures (glycosylation and protein synthesis); cell differentiation, division, and growth; targeted cell death (apoptosis); and maintaining homeostasis (water balance and metabolism). If cells lack glycans, this will affect their ability to sense their environment. Therefore, they might not recognize what food is available and needed, what toxins are blocking the system, what cells need to be built or killed for the benefit of an efficient system, or even how to maintain a healthy metabolism.

To give an example of how simply one of these processes can malfunction, let us look at protein synthesis (making protein structures). As mentioned in our chapter on epigenetics, gene expression is influenced by how we live, and how we live influences what happens to us through cell communication. Let's look a little more closely at this process. Signals are sent from the cell membrane to the nucleus to download certain codes of information in order to make something happen within the cell. A copy is made of that code of information on a messenger RNA (mRNA); then the mRNA is sent to the ribosomes to give instructions to make the proteins necessary to complete the next task of the cell. Once the proteins are put in a structure, they undergo a process called "protein folding," which allows proteins to be functional. When messages coming from the glycan structures are heard and communicated properly, proteins are made in alignment with the messages as well as the needs of the body. Glycans manage this process through molecular membrane trafficking (cellular communication at the cell membrane). Glycans also differentiate what is what in the cell and can activate molecular clearance when necessary (the process by which toxic materials are released from the cells and from the body). When any of the messages about protein folding, molecular membrane trafficking, or molecular clearance are misunderstood or unclear due to missing or insufficient glycans, this can result in misfolded proteins. Misfolded proteins, in turn, can result in cell dysfunction, tissue damage, and eventually diseases like cancer, Type II diabetes, neurological disorders, and cardiovascular disease.[7]

As I studied this subject and realized that these were merely the basic cell activities of the body, I was in awe of the magnitude and complexity of our system. Things go well for most of us, most of the time, which is amazing in itself. However, as our food is being altered and as we experience more daily stress, the demands on our physical being are becoming too much for many of us.

The Johns Hopkins University School of Medicine's Department of Biological Chemistry has studied the functions of glycans in relation to cancer, diabetes, and neurodegeneration. The results of these research efforts are beginning to transform the way the medical world understands the roles sugars play in the molecular mechanisms of disease. Through my research, I also learned that Oxford University was studying how different combinations of these glycans showed a correlation between certain glycan codes and certain diseases that are acquired through life as well as inherited. One journal article showed that changes in the level of expression of the glycans can cause abnormal glycan structure. One of the many examples given was that of autoimmune rheumatological diseases. When certain sugars are missing from the glycocalyx, it becomes difficult for the cells of the body to identify the self-cell-recognition code, and therefore the immune system begins to attack itself.[8] This is the basis for all autoimmune diseases. In this study, they found that autoimmune disease is often accompanied by a decrease in the galactosylation process. (The glycosylation process of galactose, one of the eight glycan sugars, is called galactosylation.) When this process does not result in the proper structure of a glycan code, it is referred to as altered or aberrant glycosylation, as mentioned above. Again, coming to the basic principle: if the glycan structure has not been made properly, it cannot function properly.

Caring for Our Immune Systems

Early in my nursing career, we were introduced to a new disease called AIDS, caused by the HIV virus. Nobody knew what it was, and there was a lot of fear around it. Similar to the first few months of the Covid-19 pandemic, we didn't have a test to find out if someone had it or not. We didn't have a clue what we were dealing with. The ward that I worked on back then cared for many AIDS patients. These patients were all very sick. Some were already dying and/or were highly contagious. Their immune systems were greatly affected, and they would get infections everywhere in their body—in their lungs, brains, skin, and hearts—and they often had high fevers. It was difficult to help when we knew so little and there was still so much fear. AIDS was only transmitted through specific contact, whereas today, viruses like Covid-19 seem in many ways stronger and more aggressive, even if they are less deadly overall. So, what can we learn? Decades of helping HIV patients have taught the medical community that those with the virus must take very good care of themselves to maintain their immune function and prevent themselves from contracting secondary infections. Now, perhaps everyone should follow that advice. Our immune system is the most powerful guardian of our physical health, and we need to support it powerfully and continually.

If you accept that we are Creators, the question arises: "What has happened to the environment, and to the world, to create such high levels of illness in the collective?" On some level, consciously or unconsciously, our choices have weakened our immune systems. What is disease really showing us? Just like with our bodies, we need to have a strong environment that can protect and defend itself. We and nature are one. When we are out of balance, we affect nature, and when nature is out of balance, it affects us. The law of cause and effect works both ways.

Since our cells execute every task our bodies require to live, creating boundaries and providing protection via our immune system is vital for not simply surviving, but ultimately thriving. As we grow in consciousness, we learn that we can ask for more from life—in fact, that as humans we are capable of more. In order to go to a level of thriving, we must first master the basic needs of our physical body. We must master care for our own systems—most importantly, our immune system.

THE IMMUNE SYSTEM AND GLYCANS

Interestingly, the immune system is dependent on glycans for the protection of cell systems and the entire body. As we've learned, glycans communicate with everything in our bodily environment. They are basically the eyes, ears, and sensing ability of our cells. They help us identify every player in the body and instruct the cells how to behave from moment to moment. Our immune system has a natural surveillance system of its own. It is constantly monitoring our entire body every day for dangerous invaders and/or toxins. As mentioned above they are also constantly checking if all the cells belong (self-cell-recognition). In terms of immunity, glycans act like "bouncers" for our cells. Without enough glycans, cells cannot protect and defend themselves or us. There are two aspects of the immune system: the innate and the adaptive. The innate immune system is the first line of defense when new bacteria or toxins enter the body; it responds similarly whether or not the invader has been encountered before. The adaptive immune system is built over time, includes cellular memory, and can help the system respond more quickly and efficiently. For example, when Covid-19 first appeared as a new virus, our innate immune systems were activated. Today, with all the new variants, the virus does not pose the same threat as our system has already "seen" it, and our adaptive immune system has knowledge of how to deal with it and can therefore react much more quickly.

Glycans play a large role in both the innate and adaptive immune response and are essentially the communicators of the system. They are responsible for modulating the response. What do I mean by modulating? They ensure that the system responds clearly and appropriately, not too little and not too much. When the system is overstimulated, a person can experience an external threat, like allergies, or an internal threat such as autoimmune disease. Autoimmunity occurs when glycans are insufficient or unable to identify who's who in the body; as mentioned above, because of this confusion, the immune system attacks the body's own cells. If they do this in the thyroid, it is called Hashimoto's Thyroiditis; if this takes place in the joints, it is called arthritis. What is important to understand is that it is the same problem but only in different areas of the body. On the other hand, when the immune system is "asleep" or underreacting, we have an increased risk of infection or cancer development.

Glycans not only modulate the immune response, but they also act as a decoy and can protect the cells from invaders that pose a danger to them. When glycans are abundant in the system, they can bind to the pathogen and then transport it out of the system. When glycans are not abundant, the cell membrane and signaling responses are weakened, which leaves the cell more susceptible to invaders.

The immune system is composed of many different players that must work together for the benefit of an efficient system. The glycans are vital for ensuring that communication is quick, clear, and coherent. Leukocytes (neutrophils) help kill bacteria and viruses and are the first line of defense when there is a problem. They are also integral to cleaning up inflammatory responses. Macrophages help identify bacteria and viruses, engulf and digest them, also cleaning up inflammatory responses, and call for T-cell help when necessary. T-cells are known as "killer cells" that kill infected or cancerous cells in their efforts to keep the body healthy. Then, there are the B-cells, which create antibodies from proteins, are involved in cell memory, and can help eliminate and neutralize recurrent pathogens and/or toxins. There are also helper T-cells that are necessary in the adaptive immune responses. And finally, there are the epithelial cells that provide a protective barrier by controlling the body's ability to secrete, absorb, and excrete.

To summarize: chronic inflammation is a sign that the players are not working well together, and that the system of communication in general has broken down.

Glycans also play a key role in identifying and killing cancer cells. Cancerous cells are basically cells that have gone rogue. They have forgotten who they are and what their task is in the body. The body, through its immune system, is programmed to identify and kill these cells via programmed cell death, known as apoptosis. When glycans are not abundant, the cell membrane and signaling responses are weakened, leaving cells more susceptible to invaders or the "forgetting" that leads to cancerous growth. Glycans also manage a process called "cell adhesion," in which cells of a certain type tend to bind together to stay where they belong. When cells do not bind well together, they can migrate to other areas of the body. If this migration involves cancerous cells, it is known as metastasis. When enough glycans are present they can prevent the migration of cancer cells to other parts of the body.

The ability of the immune system to modulate the immune response is the responsibility of the glycans. The stronger one's immune system is, the more easily it will be able to contain cancer cells from growing and metastasizing. A balanced immune system is important for our health and imperative for our wellness. Although the body needs all nutrients for health, without the glycans conducting the orchestra the system cannot function coherently.

VIRUSES AND OUR IMMUNE SYSTEM

If there is one thing I have come to know in my quest to understand optimal health, it is that everything in the body has a purpose and is also playing out in the duality of our human reality. Viruses are no different. Just like bacteria, they can play different roles in the body. Some will play the "good guys," and others the necessary "bad guys."

Many scientists are still struggling to understand the true nature and function of viruses. And, it's no wonder: researchers estimate that there are more viruses on this planet than there are stars in the universe, and that viruses outnumber bacteria ten to one.[9] Much is still to be discovered about how viruses work, but what is clear is that each person has their own unique individual collection, which, more often than not, serves their individual health and well-being. The human virome is the total collection of viruses in and on the body.

Viruses are microscopic carriers of information. They transmit either through DNA or RNA. Both DNA and RNA are essentially bringing and transmitting information to ensure connection, communication, and evolution. If viruses are information, they influence and serve humanity, as their influence on the human genome will go on for generations. Researchers at the Smithsonian Institution noted in one article that, "Most of the genetic information on Earth probably resides within them, and viruses are important for transferring genes between different species, increasing genetic diversity and ultimately enhancing evolution and the adaptation of various organisms to new environmental challenges."[10] From that perspective, we can conclude that viruses ensure that we continue to upgrade our DNA and evolve.

Viruses work by entering a cell, hijacking that cell's DNA, and replacing that DNA with its own message. This influences the fate of the cell. While it's easy to assume that this is a negative process, science is showing us that the effects can be quite positive in the long run. Paolo Mita, studying viruses in the genome at the NYU School of Medicine in New York, said, "When you look at [viruses'] role in one human lifespan, most likely if they are mobilized there are going to be negative effects ... on the other hand, if you are looking across time, these elements are a powerful force of evolution."[11] For instance, at the University of Utah, it was discovered that a retrovirus in our human genome infected our ancestors somewhere between 45 and 60 million years ago. That viral invasion switched on a gene called AIM2, which directly set off a cascade of information in the body to improve overall immune response.[12]

If all parts of us and our environment play a role in our health and well-being, either by supporting or bringing long-term balance to the system, then viruses as well as bacteria, fungi, and even parasites can ultimately benefit and keep our entire systems in check. However, there is a delicate balance between all these players. If any one of them becomes too dominant or aggressive, they can disrupt this balance and cause illness. The health of the microbiome influences the health of the virome, and vice versa. Additionally, viruses seem to work together and influence each other as well as the host. An imbalanced system can allow deadly viruses or opportunistic bacteria to create chaos and disease.

Glycans also play a role in how well we recognize virulent viruses, how quickly we respond to them, and how fast we clean up the damage caused by them. Glycans coat both the linings of the cell's membrane as well as the linings around the viruses; through these membranes, the cell and the virus communicate. Viruses can alter their glycan coat to attach to the cell membrane and then infect the cell. The glycans in this process also begin the process of triggering innate and adaptive immunity. If the immune system is strong, the host cell can recognize the virus and trigger an effective immune response. However, if the immune system's cell communication is weak, the virus can evade detection and clearance.

Many viruses, particularly retroviruses like HIV, seem to hang out

1 Your Creator Matrix

in the genome waiting for the immune system to weaken so they can start replication. Other viruses, like Epstein-Barr and human papillomavirus (HPV), can influence and even stimulate genetic mutation, pushing cells toward becoming cancerous. This is why the efficiency of our immune system matters, even when we aren't actively sick. Our lifestyle choices, coupled with our unique bio-individuality, may leave us vulnerable to more severe viral attacks. This supports epigenetics; what we choose can influence which genes get turned on, and which genes get turned off—whether that turning on and off is directed by our own body or an invading virus.

While much is still unknown, it's clear that good self-care is foundational to wellness regardless of our current virome. As we learned in previous chapters, it is important not only to care for our bodies, but also to trust and love them; by doing so we remain in high-frequency emotions, rather than allowing ourselves to get caught up in the lower-frequency emotion of fear, for example.

Brain Health and Glycans

A great deal has changed over the years about our understanding of how the brain works.

The brain is "mission control" for the entire body and nervous system. It is responsible for controlling the spinal cord and peripheral nervous system, memory, mental abilities, moods, hormones, energy levels, digestion, and other bodily functions.

When I was a young nurse, I was taught that once we lose our brain cells, there is no way to get them back. However, in practice, I saw time and time again people regaining their original neurological abilities after suffering serious physical brain traumas. Today, the emerging science of neurogenesis is showing us that it's possible to not only rejuvenate our current brain cells, but also to create new ones. In fact, one study estimated that 700 new neurons are added in the adult hippocampus every day.[13] Also, through brain scans, we can see that the brain can repair itself based on how we use it, what we eat, how we think, how we process emotions, and how and when we exercise. For brain health, the expression "use it or lose it!" should be our mantra for life!

As we explored in previous chapters, "neuroplasticity" refers to the ability of the brain to create new neural pathways. As it continues to reorganize itself, the brain can change its structure and ultimately its function. To grasp how the brain works and changes, it is important to understand neurons and synapses. The process of making new neurons is known as neurogenesis. Every time we learn something new, we create new neural networks with neurons and synapses. Neurons are brain cells that connect through synapses. Synapses are strengthened when we continue to use the same pathways by thinking the same thoughts over and over again. When we stop using these pathways and cease thinking certain thoughts continuously, the synapse is weakened.

Stress has a powerful influence on our brain and mental health. I learned the true power of this after recovering from my postpartum depression. As I shared earlier, I had a burnout after giving birth, and what turned things around for me was learning to meditate. Meditation helped to "declutter" my brain. It also helped me to become more focused and positive. As neuropsychologist Donald Hebb quipped, "Neurons that fire together, wire together." What I learned from my burnout experience is that my brain was depleted and cluttered with negative thoughts and unprocessed emotions. These factors were contributing to the anxiety and panic attacks that I was suffering from.

During my journey of recovery, I met a psychiatrist who explained that when the brain is under stress for a prolonged period of time, the neurons cannot "fire together." Instead, there is confusion and chaos, which results in a depletion of neurotransmitters. This can cause a "slowing" of the brain and a change in its biochemistry. This is why, in depression and anxiety disorders, people may not be able to get rid of negative thoughts. He explained that everyone can have negative thoughts, but when the brain is working properly, they do not completely take over.

Eating healthy food is a major factor in the health of our brain.

Glycans play a significant role in all brain functions because they make connections happen between cells. Every thought and memory retrieval requires proper cell signaling. Glycans support synaptic efficiency between neurons, which helps us with memory, focus, attention, clarity, and our ability to make new connections. Glycan availability also helps with the proper formation of cells in the brain, and with our ability to build proper neural structures that can transmit light and information.

We also need glycans to clean up toxins in the brain. Many neurodegenerative diseases involve the misfolding and accumulation of abnormal toxic protein. Alzheimer's disease, the most common form of dementia, is a disorder now understood to be caused by a buildup of misfolded proteins known as amyloid plaque and tau. Remember, glycans help proteins to fold properly! JC Spencer, CEO of The Endowment for Medical Research, concludes, "Correct the protein folding problem and you correct a wide range of problems." Researchers all over the world are trying to discover the ways in which glycans direct proteins. As we learn more about this process, we will understand more of the reasons why the body breaks down.

A recent study by Johns Hopkins University, published in *Neuroscience News,* explains that "cleaning up the brain from toxins (amyloid plaque and tau) is the job of the brain's immune system ... when cleanup is impaired, Alzheimer's disease is more likely to occur."[14] Medical researchers performed "reverse engineering" on five people who had died of Alzheimer's disease, and found that glycans could play an important role. In these five people, they found an overabundance of the receptor CD33 on microglia cells. It was noted in the study that these connector molecules were glycans. Microglia cells make up approximately 10 percent of the brain and are the most common immune cells of the central nervous system. They support cognition and are responsible for the repair of tissue damage and inflammation of the brain. They are also involved in many disease processes such as strokes and infections. Ronald Schnaar, PhD, Professor of Pharmacology at the Johns Hopkins University School of Medicine and director of the laboratory that led the study, stated, "Receptors are not active on their own. Something needs to connect with them to block microglia from cleaning up these toxic proteins in the brain." Their conclusion was that glycoproteins may be connecting with more CD33 receptors in Alzheimer's patients than in those with healthy brains, thus limiting the brain's ability to clean up harmful proteins.[15] This suggests that perhaps the glycoproteins could be misfolded or unable to "see" what needs to be done to clean up the system.

The glycan that has the greatest influence on the brain is sialic acid. It is important in all neural cell interactions. The brain has the highest concentration of sialic acid (also known as N-acetylneuraminic acid) in the body. This sugar usually occupies the terminal position of the glycan chain and is vitally important in the cell-to-cell communication process. As a labor and delivery nurse, I saw the power of breastfeeding for newborns; when I began studying glycans, I discovered that they were in human breast milk. I then realized the connection between breastfeeding and a baby's strong immune system and brain development.

Studies have shown that the ingestion of glycans improves cognition, perception, and memory. One study was conducted by Howard University in Washington, D.C. on sixty-two healthy young adults. Participants were given one tablespoon of glycans forty-five minutes before performing cognitive tests. Those who received glycans showed significantly improved "visual discrimination and working memory" over the control group.[16] With neurological diseases manifesting more frequently and in increasingly younger populations, it is imperative that we appreciate how glycoscience can improve our brain health. Learning to manage our stress and improve lifestyle habits, and eating more glycans, can be a strong step toward improving our brain health and vitality.

STEM CELLS AND GLYCANS

Maintaining a state of health and wellness is about being able to rejuvenate. We make a million cells per second, and the health of our cells will determine how we age. During the last few years, scientists have learned a great deal about stem cells and the important part they play in this process. It is now known that it's possible for the body to stay youthful and healthy by harnessing the power of stem cells. Not only have scientists been working on using stem cells to cure diseases, but they are also beginning to understand the power of activating them for long-term health.

The human body is made up of many different types of cells. Stem cells are the foundational cells of the body and are unspecified. They are instructed by the body to divide and differentiate. Once they are differentiated, they have a specific function in a specific part of the body—i.e., pancreatic cells, brain cells, liver cells, etc.

As we age, however, our stem cells' ability to regenerate declines. As adults, we have stem cells throughout the body; these remain inactive until either a disease or tissue injury. When repairs are needed, stem cells are differentiated (activated) to become whatever cells are needed to restore the health of the system. Glycans play a critical role in stem cell differentiation. Basically, they direct and oversee the process, and ensure that stem cell differentiation is carried out properly. Glycans do this through the process of cell signaling we explored in the previous section.

In the field of regenerative medicine, stem cell therapy is being researched as an alternative to organ transplantation. Other research is focusing on increasing the amount of stem cells in the body for health. One way to enhance stem cell function is through nutrition and lifestyle choices. By eating more nutrient-dense foods and/or supplementing with missing nutrients, it is possible to optimize the conditions of our cells for rejuvenation and repair. Specific plants like brown seaweed and aloe contain glycans that have been documented to support this process. All eight glycans in general improve cell communication, cell adhesion, and modulation of the immune system, and can help stem cells to develop properly (differentiate) and remain in the correct location in the body. A study that was conducted on the daily ingestion of fucoidans (a sulfated polysaccharide derived from brown seaweed that contains three glycans) in mice found that fucoidans helped prevent stem cell death by making subjects better able to modulate apoptosis (cell death).[17] Another study showed that ingesting fucoidans increased the number of stem cells in study subjects.[18]

Glycans and the Creator Matrix

I constantly feel wonder and amazement at how beautifully the body works. Studying and learning about glycoscience brings me constant excitement and hope for our understanding of the complexity, and also the simplicity, of coherent connection and communication on a cellular level, and how these factors support a healthy system.

It has been well established that healthy cells have many glycoproteins on the cell membrane, whereas less-healthy cells have fewer. In the future, it may be possible to ascertain the number of glycoproteins on the surface of every cell as a biomarker for health and wellness. When you look at the billions of potential configurations such communication entails, it's no wonder glycans have been so challenging to study! However, researchers are making progress. In a study titled, "Sugars Communicate through Water: Oriented Glycans Induce Water Structuring," researchers were able to show how glycans influenced the water in and around a cell. The glycan antennas imposed an "ordering" on the water. The way in which the glycans structured the water impacted the cell's ability to interact with all molecules in its vicinity. The study authors concluded that glycans are "multi-antennary structures" that seem to transcend the physical world as we currently understand it.[19]

I am convinced that our children will be taught this science as part of their basic education in the near future. As new tech companies make headway into breaking the glycan codes, others will use this knowledge more practically. For example, in agriculture, this science is already being applied to food, and aims to help us grow food in such a way that it contains a sufficient amount of the structural sugars (macronutrients) we so desperately need. The question will then become, "Do we want to ingest these sugars in a natural way, or take a synthetic version?" From my research, I am convinced that glycans as they exist in nature are superior and are non-toxic for our bodies.

We are only beginning to understand the true impact of what this area of knowledge will bring humanity. As interesting as the emerging research is, glycoscience has implications far beyond cellular health. I am certain that understanding cell communication and connections will bring a new dimension to our awareness and consciousness of how our body, mind, and spirit work together to create well-being. As we learned previously in this book, the communication network between body, mind, and spirit is essential to our ability to be Creators. Glycans are a significant part of that picture.

Chapter Summary

- Healing is not fixing what is broken but reconnecting on all levels of body, mind, and spirit. To heal is to become whole, to reconnect and find oneself again.

- Our cells communicate constantly. Cell-to-cell connection and communication is important to the wellness of our whole being. Glycans are the basis for cell-to-cell communication. They act like antennas that are responsible for our cells' ability to communicate. Messages are sent every second in real time at the cell level based on the needs of the body, mind, and spirit.

- Glycoscience is the study of glycans (sugars) and how they function in the body. Eight glycans are responsible for cell communication: glucose, galactose, mannose, fucose, xylose, glucosamine, galactosamine and sialic acid (neuraminic acid). They look like a forest on the cell surface membrane.

- Glycans play roles in almost every biological process and are involved in every major disease. Elimination of any single major class of glycans from an organism results in death.

- Glycans transmit information with the help of a universal electromagnetic field. This is a multidimensional process that can be influenced by all fields of existence: physical, mental, emotional, and spiritual. Glycans communicate with everything in their environment: nutrients (lectins), hormones, enzymes, viruses, bacteria, toxins, antibodies, and other microorganisms.

- Glycans communicate to protect, nourish, clean, and receive information in order to carry out cellular tasks that align with the needs of the whole organism at any given moment. Glycans play a role in protein folding, molecular membrane trafficking, molecular clearance, immune response modulation, self-cell-recognition, brain functions, stem cell differentiation, etc.

- Healthy cells have many glycoproteins on the cell membrane. In order to transmit accurate messages, it is essential that the glycan structures are made well. When the communication of the cells is clear, the cells can function easily and coherently, and the body can function optimally.

- In glycoscience (glycobiology) the focus is on glycans in terms of disease process and pharmacology. In nutritional glycoscience the focus is on the glycans in their natural state in food. Glycans should be found in many of our fruits and vegetables, however modern agricultural methods and food processing have eliminated many glycans from most foods we eat.

- We can optimize the conditions of our cells for rejuvenation and repair by increasing our glycan intake through nutrition: eating more nutrient-dense foods, choosing organic food sources, and natural (non-synthetic) supplementation of missing nutrients.

- Understanding cell communication and connections will bring new dimensions to our awareness and consciousness of how our body, mind, and spirit work together to create well-being, which is essential to our ability to be Creators.

Chapter Ten

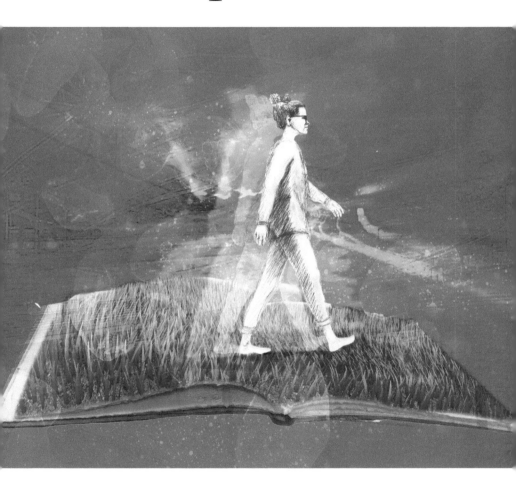

*How is your consciousness
directing your biology?*

"Our greatest human adventure is the evolution of consciousness. We are in this life to enlarge the soul, liberate the spirit, and light up the brain."

- **Tom Robbins**

CHAPTER TEN

The Biology of Consciousness

O ur consciousness will influence our body and all biological systems, just like our physical reality will affect our consciousness. Learning how to use our consciousness to direct our biology is also how we will master our Creator Matrix.

So, how is your consciousness directing your biology? I understood this concept more easily when I changed the words around. As I reorganized the words, two new concepts emerged: "our consciousness within our biology," and "our consciousness incarnated in our biology." In Latin, "incarnate" means "in the flesh."[(1)] When we look at our Creator Matrix, we see our mind-spirit complex coming into physical form through our bodies.

To more deeply understand the idea of our Creator Matrix, we will now explore the connection between the spiritual and physical as we begin to integrate the totality of our learning in this book.

The New Age: Connecting Beyond the Physical

Theologians, philosophers, and channelers have been speaking of a "new time" for years. Others have written songs, directed movies, and written books about what this new time would look like. Some have called it the Age of Aquarius, The New Age, The Shift, Spiritual Leap in Consciousness, The Great Expansion, Evolutionary Jump, The End Times, The Awakening, and The Acceleration of Evolution. Others have described it in terms of an energy shift—for example, moving from linear energy to expansional energy, new energy, and/or multidimensional energy.

One thing is clear, however: we are moving beyond our linear, physical perspective.

I began to awaken to this reality of a new time in the early 2000s. During that period, my spiritual teacher, Titia Licht, recommended many books for me to read by channelers who were leading the way in the shift that was already underway. Many lightworkers in my community were also waking up then. I decided to unify and support this group by holding regular meetings at my house. Most of us were helping people heal in our own unique ways. During these meetings, we shared information and experiences about the changes that were taking place. We recognized that these changes would accelerate even more as we drew closer to the year 2012. The most wonderful part of acknowledging the shift in consciousness at that time was being able to share it with like-minded people. These meetings gave us hope that we were not alone, as well as the courage to bring many new ideas to humanity.

The awakening process has been intensifying dramatically since 2020. This will continue as we are now on the brink of the new world.

Both in spiritual circles and outside of them, many are looking to science to explain the changes and phenomena we are experiencing. As you've seen in this book, quantum science, epigenetics, glycoscience, and neuroscience all offer their own answers and connections. Although consciousness is always adapting and evolving, our physical world is also rapidly changing; our recent quantum leap in technology alone illustrates how significant these changes are. Our "inner world" of consciousness has always been directing the changes we see in our physical reality. Now, we are simply becoming aware of this connection as we awaken to our Creatorship.

Day by day, we seem to get a greater overview and understanding of the new world we are creating. Unlike a fish in a fishbowl who sees only its reflection, we can now begin to see outside the lines of our limited three-dimensional container. Some of us are beginning to feel the boundaries of our world changing, almost as if time itself is changing. We have become more in touch with ourselves energetically, understanding that we *are* energy and that we have an energetic field that impacts everything inside and around us—that there is a direct relationship between our inner world and what shows up in our outer world.

In the past, we operated from a limited set of possibilities. However, as our consciousness expands, so too does our access to greater potentialities. Our present-day reality is changing, and the base of the change is that energy is working holographically—meaning, across many dimensions simultaneously—and thereby enhancing our ability to access and utilize our true human potential. Quantum research is already shaking the very foundation of what we know and what is familiar. This makes the awakening process uncomfortable at times, but also exhilarating.

Our awakening, as we've explored, involves the release and cleaning of old programs, belief systems, traumas, and emotional karmic memories that have been stored in the DNA. Once a person has "cleaned up" their old patterns and has gone through the process of accepting and releasing past blockages, they can embrace a new, more conscious way of living.

By living in the "now" moment, we can co-create with the Universal Field (Prime Creator). It is important to remember that when our thoughts and emotions are focused on the past or the future, we have no access to this powerful connection with the Universal Field. This field is only active and accessible to us when we are consciously interacting with it in the here and now. Many of us—out of fear, anxiety, and programmed patterns—play out dramas over and over again in our minds. We become stuck in the thoughts, emotions, and storylines that have occurred in the past and/or potentially may unfold in the future. When we are living in the past or future, we have no power to be a Creator.

What we must remember is this: we can change everything and anything by *realizing* that we can! Being a Creator requires us to learn to live in the present moment, release and empty our Creator Matrix, consciously and biologically connect our intentions to the field, and trust the process. As we make our intentions, we can fill our Creator Matrix with positive energy that mirrors the creation we wish to bring into our reality. It is important to remain present and feel the highest possible expression of this creation. The best way to describe this feeling is as a state of expansion or "exhilarating wholeness." Remember, we will feel this expansion in our hearts, as the heart has the largest electromagnetic field of any organ in the body. As we master this process, we will begin to experience many positive changes in our lives.

When we can connect our thoughts, emotions, and intentions through our integrated Creator Matrix to the Universal Field, we can send and receive messages. In this way, we are living multidimensionally. When I experience this personally, I feel a warm sensation and expanding frequencies around the center of my chest, and an exuberant feeling in my heart as I connect to my intuitive knowing and "sixth sense" abilities. When my senses are heightened, I can see what I could never see before, hear what I could never hear before, and feel what I could never feel before. This interactive process leaves me both exhilarated and peaceful with an overall feeling of wholeness and completeness. In this expanded state, I can open myself to receive messages from the Universal Field, and what seem like miracles and/or synchronicities start showing up.

I once heard Dr. Joe Dispenza say, "How can you 'want' when you are whole?" I understand this wholeness to be our future as we begin to embrace a multidimensional existence.

Let's look at a few examples of our shift into quantum reality.

The first realization is that there *is* a quantum reality, and that we can access it. The second realization is that we can interact with this quantum energy, thereby entering a new reality and reaping the benefits of becoming more whole. And finally, to do this more easily and naturally, we will need to refine our abilities by consciously practicing.

My first experiences of connecting with quantum energy occurred when I started helping people heal with my hands through high-light frequency. Many years ago, I was at home in Amsterdam when my son called me from Washington, D.C.. He was feeling very sick. Although I accessed the quantum field regularly through my Reconnective Healingwork, this was the first time I had used the technique without being in physical proximity to the recipient. I wondered if this frequency healing would indeed be able to transcend space and time to connect to his aura and neutralize his imbalance. I asked him to please lie down so I could connect to his aura, just like I did with my in-person clients. I immediately felt a chaotic frequency in his aura. I began to use the techniques I had been practicing and, to both of our amazement, he began to feel better almost immediately. Today I can access this field instantly, helping others outside the linear three-dimensional reality.

Another clue that we are connected to the quantum field is when we start receiving messages and information at all times of the day or night. Multidimensional reality has no regard for linear time; hence, information will often come flooding in and wake us up in the middle of the night! When I was writing my Health and Wellness Coaching training course in 2017, I would often be woken up to write down information for the course. I was annoyed at first and tried to resist it because it was disturbing my sleep, but after a while I began to understand that, if I didn't write it down, it would disappear by morning. It was literally a flash of light containing information, available only at that moment.

When I was a nurse, many people shared with me that they had had dreams or realistic visions of someone dying at a particular moment, only to find out later that the person had, indeed, died at that same moment. My ability to connect to those on the "other side" has markedly increased since I began working with the quantum field. For example, I can think of someone—my mother, for instance—and tune into her essence, much like turning the knob on an old-school radio to find a radio station. Every time I did this "tuning in," I would receive information that was valuable to me and could guide me at that moment. And, as I've shared elsewhere in this book, this ability also allowed me to connect to the Archangel Michael while on vacation in Florida.

Through my work, I have seen that the children being born onto the planet at this time seem to have easier and more streamlined access to these multidimensional realms. More of their DNA has been cleared of the old blockages, and their bodies can contain more light and information at the cellular level. This affects and increases their perception multidimensionally. They seem to be more connected to their hearts, which brings more "knowingness." For those of us who are older, the shroud of illusion is beginning to thin, but it will take practice and effort for us to learn to access the quantum field and its light information with ease.

Connecting to the quantum field will impact our power as Creators tremendously. It will not only increase our powers to heal, but also our powers to manifest in the physical reality. We will become more aware of our thoughts, emotions, and decisions as we begin to align our body, mind, and spirit to the field of infinite possibilities. When we practice this alignment, our hearts can leap for joy as we attract our dreams into our reality. Understanding how our energetic system affects the material world, and how our thoughts, words, actions, and decisions affect our physical reality, we will do away with the linear, reductionist methods of healing so common to Western medicine and approach the idea of healing from a holistic, holographic viewpoint. This will also extend to the unique root causes of disease: what for one person was caused primarily by emotional traumas could be caused by physical or environmental factors in another person. In order to create optimal wellness, we can and should examine *all* factors that influence disease and health, wellness, and wholeness.

In other words, we need to look at where biology and consciousness intersect.

Involution and Evolution

Until now, we have been exploring physics, particularly quantum physics, to understand the scientific base for our reality. In order to understand the connection between the spiritual and physical more deeply, let's look at the difference between quantum physics and metaphysics.

Physics is the study of the interactions between matter and energy. Quantum physics looks at the role of the quanta (subatomic particles), how we interact with them, and how they behave; the actual science of the quantum.

To understand the interaction more clearly between the spiritual and physical, we can look to metaphysics. Meta means "beyond." Thus, metaphysics means "beyond the physical," and is more of a philosophical study of the reasons for our existence than a "hard" science. Metaphysics is defined as, "the branch of philosophy that studies the foundational nature of reality, [including] questions about the nature of consciousness."[2]

We have been compartmentalizing the sciences for generations. We have adopted highly linear, reductionist views and have tended to look at everything separately. However, the new energy is holistic, holographic, and multidimensional; therefore, it is time to integrate all of our "separated" knowledge, recognize its connectedness, and adopt a more holistic perspective that includes both physical (physics-based) and metaphysical perspectives. Humanity has made significant technological advancements in the last few hundred years, and most especially since the Industrial Revolution, and this has been mirroring our spiritual development. It is not possible to have one without the other; that isn't how consciousness works. Consciousness directs our biology just like we, as Creators, are directing all aspects of our Creator Matrix.

Theologians, philosophers, and scholars have tried for eons to look at the connections between consciousness and our physical reality. Many have been searching for answers to how consciousness actually began. Many hold different and unique belief systems about why we as spiritual beings are having this physical experience. No one person holds the complete truth; and the more we know the more we realize we don't know. To go a bit deeper in our understanding of the metaphysical philosophy of consciousness or the nature of reality, let's look at the process of both involution and evolution.

Many spiritual leaders look to mysticism to help understand the mechanisms of involution and evolution. Mysticism is defined as, "a belief in the existence of realities beyond perceptual or intellectual apprehension that are directly accessible by subjective experience."[3] In other words, mysticism helps us to understand that we cannot perceive everything with our senses. There is much that we cannot explain, and that science has not been able to either; but that doesn't mean that these unexplainable things are imaginary, or that they don't exist.

When we reflect on possibilities that could have initiated our experience here on Earth, we are often struck with the inexplicable aspects involved. Many masters and spiritual teachers suggest that involution, at the highest essence of expression, is represented by Universal Source energy manifesting itself in increasingly dense matter, including the physical reality we occupy here on Earth. Perhaps at one time there was only light in the universe. There was no contrast, duality, or density. Perhaps we, as light beings, wanted to experience existence in a more physical reality. Hence, density and darkness were created. Involution is the process of the descent from spirit into physicality—the descent toward denser and denser forms of matter. Imagine that this experience we are having in matter, and perhaps have had for eons, is only for the purpose of spirit experiencing itself in increasingly denser states. As people are on different levels of evolutionary paths, some may not yet have wondered where they came from or question what they have been told about our origins. Others are baffled by such existential questions their entire lives.

Once consciousness has explored the densest states or realms of existence, it begins its process of evolution or ascension.

As involution is the process of the descent of spirit into denser forms of matter. Evolution is the ascension into lighter forms of beingness. Evolution can be defined as, "a gradual process in which something changes into a different and usually more complex or better form."[4] This suggests that humanity is on an ever-accelerating speed train where the passengers (the inhabitants of Earth) continue to blossom into more complex and ultimately better versions of themselves. If we agree that we are all Creators, and that anything that we can think or imagine we can essentially become, we begin to see that our current spiritual evolution will eventually help us rise to our full potential. I find it hopeful that we are evolving toward a different kind of world, one where each of us is more in touch with who we are, and with the higher expression of our true essence.

Involution and evolution are counterforces that have a ripple effect through all of eternity. Descending from spirit into matter helps us become more conscious of all aspects of reality. As we ascend from denser states of matter, we gain an appreciation of these different expressions of consciousness. It's a deep spiritual journey.

Eventually, as many of us try to understand our spiritual purpose, we may find it comforting to know that we are evolving spiritually. Life, as an experience, makes more sense with a spiritual purpose. A great number of my clients have woken up to a more spiritual focus after experiencing life-altering events such as an accidents, illnesses, divorce, or other trauma. Many have shared with me that they now feel gratitude for those experiences, as they brought them closer to their divine essence and purpose. It is as if they were stuck on the wrong timeline, and the incident or trauma realigned them with their true reason for being here. This is the essence of connecting spiritually: a growth into our own inner knowingness, and a deeper connection to that which is beyond our ability to understand and perceive.

As a nurse, I was often shocked by the innate power and awareness of those who were well-connected spiritually. One day, I walked into one of my patient's rooms, and although she was sitting up and looked happy and cheerful, she said to me, "Today will be my death day." I didn't understand how she could say this; severely depressed patients did, on occasion, succumb to sudden death, but this woman was responding well to her therapy. Yet, true to her prediction—or perhaps her decision—she did in fact pass on that day, just as my shift was ending. I watched her transition to another world in just a few hours. I was always awed by my patients who showed such a strong spiritual consciousness and inner strength during such difficult transitions.

We Are the Quantum Field

In the Universal Field, everything is connected, and nothing exists independently. Without our ability to connect, life would not exist, and there would be no consciousness. In fact, I would go so far as to say that consciousness *is* connection! As we grow to understand that we are connected to everything, this reality of being part of the quantum field becomes self-evident. Our ability to connect will help us integrate with all dimensions of existence and ultimately become more conscious and able to direct our physical reality.

Epigenetics and glycoscience are helping us to understand how everything is connected and how it all functions at the cellular level. Quantum physics helps us understand how electromagnetic fields govern those connections. As we awaken to a new "biology of consciousness," we are beginning to understand just how entwined the physical, mental, and spiritual aspects of our being truly are. In Chapter Nine, we introduced glycoscience, and learned how important the concepts of connection and disconnection are to our cellular health and well-being. In earlier chapters, we explored the concept of connection and disconnection in terms of the Yang/Yin Cycle. As we begin a new creation, we use yang energy. Throughout the creative process we will have thoughts and emotions that relate to the story we experience. These thoughts and emotions will need to be digested, integrated, felt, and released. It is important to take the time to go inward, and this is the yin cycle. Very often in our busy lives, we fail to take the time to process what has happened to us. We are not the story, yet we often get stuck in the emotions of our story. In this state, before digestion and assimilation are complete, we can feel disconnected from ourselves and experience a feeling of fragmentation. "Becoming" requires us to have both the courage to create, and the courage to digest, release, and integrate what the experience has brought us and how it has changed us. As we look at who we have become with love and acceptance, we can connect to a feeling of wholeness. This process of "becoming" will continue for eternity, because we are eternal, and our consciousness is forever evolving.

These principles of connection and disconnection are constantly being repeated on all levels of existence—physical, mental, emotional, and spiritual. Learning how to reconnect to all of these levels will have a ripple effect on our health and on the universe as a whole. As we become more interconnected, we will grasp that we are sovereign, powerful beings who function holistically within the framework of our Creator Matrix of body, mind, and spirit, living within and connected at all levels to the quantum field.

QUANTUM CONNECTION, COMMUNICATION, AND FREQUENCY

When physicists dig down into the building blocks of matter, they observe that the smaller these building blocks get, the more mysterious the universe looks. Subatomic units, like quarks and gluons, behave more like waves than particles. Deep down, the very essence of all that surrounds us, and all that is inside us, is energy, not matter.

As we have explored in previous chapters, we are energy beings, and our energy vibrates at a frequency. Our frequencies determine our connections with the people, things, and frequencies we interact with. The new scientific revolution is showing us that our thoughts and emotions play an active, even determinant, role in determining our frequency, and therefore in the life situations we encounter and in the outcomes of our actions. What we do, think, feel, and eat every day contributes to creating our experience, beginning at the level of our DNA.

Everything in the universe is connected in a multidimensional manner through the quantum field. Some people call this field Source,

God, or Universal intelligence, to name but a few; regardless of how you prefer to relate to it, its power and potential are indeed limitless. Quantum entanglement shows us how two particles can be in relationship to each other (entangled with each other). These two particles communicate with each other and hold mirroring information, even when they are physically separated by miles or light years. We, as humans, have our own individual fields that can connect and communicate with everything in the quantum field, including the fields of other humans. Once we understand this, we can start to use our creative abilities in a whole new way.

Within the body, all of our parts influence and affect each other. Yet, the whole is greater than the sum of its parts. Our physical body connects and communicates with our thoughts; our thoughts connect and communicate with our emotions.; our emotions and thoughts connect and communicate with the infinite quantum field. This is how we, as Creators, can influence our reality and enact change on all levels of our being. As mentioned above, we as humans are now moving from linear to expansional energy. It's like going from being a train on the tracks to a bird in flight. With our thoughts and emotions influencing our energetic fields, we need periodically to recalibrate our frequencies to make sure we don't get pulled back down into linear, disempowered thinking and lose perspective on our abilities as Creators. This not only means becoming conscious of our thoughts, emotions, and actions, but also supporting our DNA and glycans through optimal well-being practices.

Our Cells are Multidimensional

Each human cell has its own consciousness that governs its health and well-being. As explained in previous chapters, our cells receive information, nourishment, and guidance from our thoughts, emotions, food, and environment, all of which are communicated to the cell with the help of glycans and our electromagnetic fields. Our consciousness affects our cellular consciousness and vice versa. In this way, our inside world reflects our outside world, and our outside world reflects our inner one. They are connected.

We've already seen how optimal physical nutrition and well-being can support cell vitality. However, being the Creators that we are, our thoughts, emotions, and life stories impact our cellular stories as well, and that DNA can and does carry imprinted memories for generations. It is a web of circuitry that transmits information through light.

We have explored the importance of glycans to this process on a physical level. Glycans are physically multidimensional and look like crystalline branches of a tree sprouting in all directions; they are structurally complex and constantly reconfigure themselves in real time, depending on the messages they need to send or receive. They influence structure at the cellular level, and structure is function. However, the most important thing to know is that they create a *light field* of information.

In my research to understand glycans better, I became aware that glycans are sugars, and sugars are crystals. In a solid state, sugar is crystallized. Crystals hold light and information. For millennia, people have used crystals like quartz, tourmaline, or citrine to facilitate different energy experiences. Today, many of our technologies use crystals to store and transmit frequencies and information in a balanced and orderly way. Similarly, our glycans vibrate (oscillate) at different frequencies, and also in response to other frequencies. As glycans send and receive signals, they create a physical wave that communicates with electromagnetic fields.

DNA is crystalline as well. According to Linden Gledhill, a biochemist and photographer, "DNA crystals form when a double helix is suspended in liquid that evaporates. They grow in patterns dictated by the information stored within the strands. Seen in cross-polarized light, they display a mind-bending kaleidoscope of color and shape."[5]

If our cells are communicating multidimensionally, we as whole beings are also communicating multidimensionally. As we evolve and transform, our bodies are transforming too. Many scientists today are observing changes at the DNA level in their epigenetic research.

Currently, we exist using two strands of DNA, which make the double-helix shape with which we are all familiar. As we are ascending in consciousness, however, many believe that more strands are being activated; some believe that as many as twelve strands or more could be activated eventually. The inactive part of our DNA has so far been referred to as "dormant" or "junk" DNA, however as more light is entering the planet at this time, these inactive parts of our coding may have a role to play. As our DNA is activated, our physical existence at the cellular level is also changing; we are transitioning from a carbon base structure to a more crystalline base, just as carbon in the earth can be transmuted into diamonds. In this way our cells become lighter and able to carry and transmit more information.

One night not very long ago, I woke up thinking about glycans, and I saw before me a crystalline network that created a web of circuitry throughout the physical body as well as the other dimensions and densities in the quantum field. I saw that our glycans and DNA are influenced by and react to every thought we think, emotion we feel, and word we speak. I have begun referring to this phenomenon as "quantum glycobiology," a field in which we understand that the entanglement of proteins, sugars, and fats on a cellular level are not merely the basic operating system of the human body, but our most potent mechanism for creation at a whole-self and universal level. We will grow through experience to master the art of connection, knowing that we are ultimately connected to and communicating with everything in the universe, all at once. As we transition to this new reality and allow greater levels of light to influence our DNA, we will become clearer and more connected to our authentic power.

Are the new sciences of epigenetics, glycoscience, quantum physics, and consciousness the keys to connecting us to our true human potential? Is our future going to be different and more wonderful than we ever imagined? Will we transform and become more of who we really are, giving us a much greater understanding of our creative power? Imagine the magnificence of what we can become and achieve. The concept of a "superhuman" is more than a mere idea; it is our impending reality.

How Consciousness Affects Cell Function

Dr. Bruce Lipton offers a simple explanation of how our thoughts control our genes at the cell level. As we now know, our cells are coated with glycoproteins that react to signals from the environment of the cell to turn genes on and off. According to Lipton:

> *"When a cell encounters nutrients, the growth genes are activated and used.*
>
> *When a cell encounters toxins, the protection genes are activated and used.*
>
> *When a human being encounters love, the growth genes are activated.*
>
> *When a human being encounters fear, the protection genes are activated."*[6]

In order for the cell to receive nutrients and love, the cell itself must be able to recognize those things—just as it must be able to recognize toxins and fear in order to eliminate them. When the cell can clearly identify what's what in the body, there is more order, coherence, and well-being of the whole. The glycan antennas are the initial connectors and protectors of this kind of coherence in the body, and their influence can activate aspects of our DNA and the quantum field.

Many other scientists and teachers have explored the relationship between our DNA and feelings. Gregg Braden (a scientist engineer) reported on three experiments which examined this phenomenon in his book, *The Divine Matrix*, and suggested that "DNA can heal itself according to the feelings of the individual." In other words, there is connection, communication, and influence between our DNA and our feelings.

In the first experiment cited in Braden's book, quantum biologist Dr. Vladimir Poponin emptied a container and created a vacuum in it, leaving particles of light behind. When he measured the remaining photons (light) inside he found that they were, as expected, distributed randomly throughout the container. He then placed DNA inside the container and measured the photons (light) again. To his surprise, the photons were not random anymore. Instead, he found that the photons were "lined up in an ordered way and aligned with the DNA." These results showed Dr. Poponin that DNA had an effect on the photons.[7] The question then became, how did the DNA influence the light? Since light is information, and information is connected to the quantum field, there must be some kind of connection between the DNA, the light, and the field. He then removed the DNA from the container and measured it again. Amazingly, the photons remained ordered and lined up where the DNA had been. The conclusion that Dr. Poponin reached was that the physical world that we observe with our eyes was capable of affecting the non-physical world even after separation. (Although more research is needed, and Dr. Poponin's work remains controversial, I feel it is thought-provoking enough to share for the purposes of this discussion.)

The second experiment was designed for the military by Dr. Cleve Backster. White blood cells were taken from individuals as DNA samples. The participants and their DNA samples were initially placed in separate rooms from each other in the same building. Each partici-pant was then subjected to watching several video clips that would elicit different types of emotions. After monitoring the participant and the DNA sample, they observed that when the participant had a certain emotional response (measured through electrical responses), both responded identically and at exactly the same time. When they took the sample 50 miles away from the participant, the results remained the same. This result showed that this energy exists everywhere all the time and is not affected by time and space.

Anyone who has ever experienced energy healing or reiki at a dis-tance will not be shocked to hear this. As I mentioned before, when I do Reconnective Healing for my son, who lives across an ocean from me, he feels it and receives the benefits every time.

An experiment by the HeartMath Institute further describes how powerful our emotions are on our health and wellness through our DNA. The study, entitled "Local and Nonlocal Effects of Coherent Heart Frequencies on Conformational Changes of DNA," placed human placenta DNA in containers in which changes to its status and structure could be measured.[8] Twenty-eight trained researchers each received a different vial of DNA. Each researcher generated strong feelings and emotions in the vicinity of the DNA. What was discovered was that the DNA changed shape according to the emotions the researchers experienced. For example, when the researchers felt love, gratitude, and appreciation, the DNA changed its shape by becoming longer and more relaxed, and their strands unwound. When the researchers felt anger, fear, frustration, or stress, on the other hand, the DNA tightened up considerably. It became shorter, and many of the DNA codes got turned off.

The experiments above illustrate two concepts in quantum mechanics, namely nonlocality and entanglement. Nonlocality refers to how two objects can have an instant connection and knowingness of each other, even when separated by long distances, including billions of light years. Quantum mechanics shows us that nonlocality is possible due to a phenomenon known as entanglement. As mentioned above, entanglement occurs when particles behave identically to each other (become entangled), almost as a single entity, yet exist in different locations.

It is understood today that one of the signs of aging DNA is shortened telomeres and exposed chromosomes. A chromosome is a long piece of DNA. The telomere's job is to protect the ends of the chromosomes. As we age, the telomeres become shorter, frayed, and tangled. Every time a cell divides, the telomere becomes a little shorter. If the ends of the chromosomes are not protected well, they will become damaged, and the DNA codes will not be properly "downloaded."

What is the significance of all of this? Imagine if we could accelerate or slow the rate of our own aging by managing our emotions. As you've learned, we have far more power to choose our emotional state than previously understood; now, we know that the states we choose today, and every day, can and do determine our physical reality for years to come. Our very timeline can be altered by learning to manage our emotions. As we change our timelines, we can change our world.

Universal energy has an intelligence of its own. Moreover, we know that when we are connected to the quantum field, we can transcend time and space as we know it. This illustrates that we already live in a multidimensional, intelligent universe. What binds us is far more complex than we ever realized. In time, perhaps we may find more evidence of our true "magical" power.

Food is Light, and Light is Information

We have trillions of cells in our body. We make a million new cells every second. Apoptosis kills a million cells each second. Over 100,000 biochemical reactions per second instruct our cells. They communicate instructions through the frequency of light.

Professor Fritz-Albert Popp was born in Germany in 1938 and earned his PhD in Theoretical Physics. He spoke about the importance of photonic light for cell communication in the body. Cells emanate photonic light that cannot be seen with our eyes. (A photon is the smallest unit of light that exists.) All communication in the body is governed by our metabolism; metabolism is life itself. The biochemical reactions in our bodies communicate through frequencies of photonic light via the crystalline structures of the glycan networks. Photonic light is information, and information is light. As Dr. Popp wrote, "We are still on the threshold of fully understanding the complex relationship between light and life, but we can now say emphatically, that the function of our entire metabolism is dependent on light."[9]

Dr. Popp describes humans as "beings of light." He further describes light as being either coherent or incoherent.[10] Healthy cells communicate with coherent light, and diseased cells emit incoherent light. Healthy cells can expand to a higher frequency, and unhealthy cells contract and stay at a lower frequency. With coherent light, communication is clear, while incoherent light is chaotic and can cause miscommunication. The ways in which we live, and how we handle our emotions, influence the coherence of our system on a daily basis.

Dr. Popp found "that the healthiest foods had the most coherent intensity of light emissions. And of course, the opposite was true. (Junk food was almost totally devoid of biophotonic emissions.)"[11] The photonic light in our body can be replenished by certain foods. When we eat fresh, whole plants high in biophotons, we can incorporate the energy from the plants into our cells. The plants' light nourishes and replenishes the light within our cells.

Plants are not the only transmitters of light. Everything we see with our eyes, from tiny microbes viewed under a microscope to planets and stars, emits light and carries information. The density and coherence of this light impacts our bodies, thoughts, and emotions on a holistic and cellular level. Therefore, the foods we choose to put into our bodies affect the coherence or incoherence of the light information provided to our cells.

Ayurvedic medicine and Traditional Chinese Medicine (TCM), among other traditional practices, give us clues as to how we can use the light and vibration inherent in our foods to balance and replenish our body, mind, and spirit. Food in its natural state has different qualities and is composed of five different elements: ether, air, fire, water, and earth. These elements are constantly in motion and dancing with each other to make this earthly existence possible and unique. Each individual's personalized combination of these elements is described in terms of *dosha* (Ayurveda) or constitution (TCM). Research is proving what these ancient traditions have known for millennia: that each person's constitution requires different foods and experiences at different times, to keep it in harmony and balance, and to maintain the coherence of the light and information fields within their body.

NOURISHING OUR BODIES WITH LIGHT TO UPGRADE OUR BIOLOGICAL CONSCIOUSNESS

We can nourish our bodies with light through increasing the frequency of all our cells. The collective light emitted from all of our cells is called our "light body." Life force becomes strong when our light body is vibrating at a high frequency. We feel better, more balanced, calmer, and happier. We can get our light from both external sources like air, sunlight, and food, and also from the breath. Breathing is the most powerful way to activate one's light body with life force. Whenever I feel stuck or sad, I take a deep breath. This always helps. Walking in nature is also very rejuvenating, as we connect with the high frequency of Mother Earth and the plant and animal kingdoms. Absorbing sunlight through both our skin and eyes can increase our frequency, too. On a physical level, sunlight also helps to regulate our circadian rhythms of sleep; and the vitamin D we produce as a result of sun exposure helps to regulate our moods as well as our immune system. We can further increase our frequency by getting enough sleep and receiving help from energy healers. Energy medicine and new technologies are coming on the market in the Age of Aquarius to support our transition into higher-frequency states. (I will discuss this further in Chapter Twelve.)

We can also increase our light through internal sources. I have learned that the fastest way to increase my frequency is by consciously activating it myself. By consciously shifting thoughts and thought patterns, we can serve the highest versions of ourselves and the lives we came here to fulfill. I also use EFT (Emotional Freedom Technique) daily; this is a wonderful way to shift our frequency quickly. We can also learn to regulate our emotions and let go of lower-frequency emotions like shame, guilt, hate, and revenge that clutter and drag down the system. While teaching my students how to shift their emotions, I often laugh at how fast they can change their state by thinking the thought of "joy."

Our current spiritual evolution is revealing the power we have as Creators to consciously tap into our spiritual essence. We will learn to care for both our physical body and light body. As we evolve and integrate our body, mind, and spirit complex, we can instantly recharge our light body which will have a direct effect on our physical well-being. As we allow light from the Universal Field to fill all our cells and ground this light in our bodies through Mother Earth, we will rejuvenate. In the world of my childhood, we were taught to do this through prayer, chanting, and religious ceremonies. Today, I find that many people accomplish the same connection through powerful intentions, meditation, yoga, tai chi, and connecting to their heart space. When we ground our spiritual light essence into our bodies then we will notice a deeper inner peace, more harmony with ourselves and others, a more loving presence, an increased ability to be creative, more lucid dreams, and more connections to synchronicities from intentions.

People who hold belief systems of hope and optimism will start to feel that this becomes their new state of being. Ultimately, we will notice that the better version of us is showing up more often.

Making intentions, thoughts, and visualizations can be the most profound way to upgrade our biological consciousness. In the next chapter, we will look more closely at what it means to live multidimensionally, and how this shift will be humanity's greatest step toward a New Earth and an upgraded, more positive reality.

Chapter Summary

- We are all awakening to a new way of living, and an increase in our awareness and consciousness. This process is happening at different times for different people.

- Our consciousness influences our body and all biological systems, just like our physical reality affects our consciousness.

- Our inside and outside world are connected: our inside world reflects our outside world and vice versa.

- We are moving beyond our physical linear perspective, moving from linear energy to new, expansional, more holistic and multidimensional energy. Energy is working holographically—meaning, across many dimensions simultaneously—and thereby enhancing our ability to access and utilize our true human potential.

- Being a Creator requires learning to live in the present moment, releasing and emptying one's Creator Matrix, consciously and biologically connecting our intentions to the field, and trusting the process. As we make our intentions, we can learn to fill our Creator Matrix with positive energy that mirrors the creation we wish to bring into our reality.

- When we are able to connect both consciously and biologically to the Universal Field, we can send and receive messages and exist multidimensionally.

- The new energy requires us to connect to our heart, which has the largest magnetic field of any organ in the body. The heart connects us to our intuitive knowing and "sixth sense" abilities.

- The "new children" on the planet are born with easier and more streamlined access to the multidimensional realms. They are more connected to their hearts, which brings more knowingness and an increased multidimensional perception.

- The metaphysical philosophy of consciousness or the nature of reality will help to understand the interaction between the spiritual and physical more clearly.

- Involution is the process of the descent of spirit into denser forms of matter. Evolution is the ascension into lighter forms of beingness.

- We are awakening to a new "biology of consciousness." We are beginning to understand just how entwined the physical, mental, and spiritual aspects of our being truly are.

- Everything in the universe is connected in a multidimensional manner through a quantum field. We, as humans, have our own individual fields that can connect and communicate with everything in the quantum field, including the fields of other humans. Consciousness *is* connection!

- Glycans create a *light field* of information. Glycans and DNA are crystalline. Crystals hold light and information. It is a web of circuitry that transmits information through light.

- As we are ascending in consciousness our DNA will evolve from two activated strands to at least twelve activated strands. This will change our physical existence at the cellular level from a carbon base structure to a crystalline base, and our cells will become lighter and able to carry and transmit more information.

- Our physical reality for years to come—our very timeline—can be altered by learning to manage our emotions. As we change our timelines, we can change our world.

- Universal energy has infinite intelligence, and time and space as we know it can be transcended. We already live in a multidimensional, intelligent universe.

- Photonic light is important for cell communication in the body. Cells are emanating photonic light. We can replenish our photonic light body with external sources like fresh, whole plant food high in biophotons, breathing air, sunlight, walking in nature, enough sleep, energy medicine, and the help of energy healers; and through internal sources like shifting our thoughts and thought patterns, EFT, and regulating our emotions.

- As we evolve, we will learn to care for both our physical body and light body. We will be able to recharge our light body instantly with light from the Universal Field, filling all our cells and grounding this light. This will have a direct effect on our physical well-being and support our rejuvenation.

Chapter Eleven

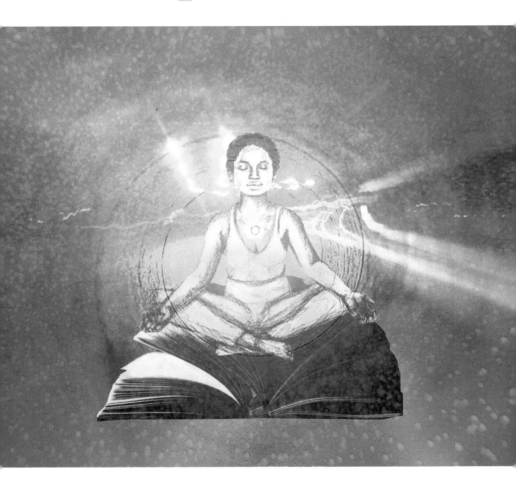

*How are you aligning and connecting
to all aspects of your Creator Matrix?*

"You exist in many levels simultaneously.
Not merely the temporal material plane of duality."

- Leland Lewis

CHAPTER ELEVEN

Quantum Reality and Multidimensional Living

L iving multidimensionally allows us to experience reality beyond the matrix of our physical form. Quantum reality is becoming our new reality, and our ability to think multidimensionally is our entry point into this quantum existence. As we adapt, we will better understand the significance between all the dimensions—body, mind, emotions, and spirit/soul—and become more aware and integrated with each of these planes of existence. Changing our perspective and making space for different thoughts can be challenging in our chaotic day-to-day lives. However, it is not possible to look at wellness and ignore the impact that our essence has on the state of wellness, and on the connections between body, mind, and spirit that make wellness possible.

The spiritual piece of the Creator Matrix is even less understood than the mind and body. Scientists, theologians, mystics, and seekers have been trying to uncover the basis for existence for eons. Many search within their faith or religion for answers, while others use psychotherapy, vision quests, or plant medicine. I was raised Catholic and spent my life searching for spiritual answers and connections through many of these avenues. I am humbled to say that the answers are still not clear. The more I know and the more I learn, the more questions I have. This fuels my desire to better understand the connection between science and our purpose as humans.

Although I am constantly amazed at the shortcomings of the scientific process when it comes to looking beyond three-dimensional reality, we continue to search for answers through the process of observation. Science is evolving, much like we are. As we gain scientific awareness it will impact our perception and consciousness growth. I also have come to realize that, while our spiritual journey can be enhanced by research and science, it is also deeply personal. We must each find and navigate our own paths with the consciousness we possess at any given moment, realizing that it can change—and will—change.

The Twelve Universal Laws of Consciousness

For millennia, humanity has been trying to understand and explain the twelve fundamental Universal Laws that govern our physical, mental, and emotional experiences (our Creator Matrix). These laws help us navigate our transition into multidimensional living. By understanding and integrating these spiritual laws, we can master our physical experience here on Earth.[1]

The Law of One

As I mentioned in Chapter Five, the first Universal Law is the Law of One. This law states that we are all connected by the universal "soup" of pure energy (the quantum field). In Chapter Ten, we learned that the origin of creation is related to the concepts of involution and evolution—in other words, that Universal Source energy seeks to experience itself, and therefore transcends from pure energy into form or matter. During this process of involution, then, the one becomes the many.

I find this exciting because, although we are all connected as one, at the same time we are individual sovereign Creator beings. Each of us evolve through lessons and experiences, developing into more complex beings with the capacity to reflect more of the consciousness of Source energy itself. How we behave, react, think, and feel are choices that reflect our internal state of being. We are all connected and are one; therefore, this internal state of being acts like a mirror to our outside reality. This works both ways as well, as we continually co-create with our environment. Nothing we allow is an accident. For example, if someone feels unsafe with others, is it just coincidence when they stop trimming the plants by their window to the point that they can no longer look out and others cannot look in? The resulting plant layer may provide a feeling of safety for them. As we evolve, we begin to see the connections between our inner and outer worlds. This mirroring process can be bumpy and uncomfortable; and it is often easier to believe that we are a victim of what shows up in our outer world and ignore the fact that we have played a part in creating it. However, if we can become neutral and non-judgmental with ourselves, we can master these changes more easily.

The Law of Attraction

The starting point for many people who are awakening has been to learn about the Law of Attraction (introduced in Chapter Six). This mirroring effect is powerful: as we create our reality, we attract what we have become. This process works through a principle of physics, simply expressed as "like attracts like." In duality, being in a negative state in our inner world can be expressed as negativity showing up in our outer world. Similarly, a positive inner state will bring more positivity into our outer reality. As we are now integrating the positive and negative (light and dark) timelines, we rise above the duality and step into our next phase of evolution.

The Law of Vibration

The next Universal Law we must master is the Law of Vibration (also mentioned in Chapter Six). This law is the foundation of the Law of Attraction. How energy vibrates determines the uniqueness of everything. Remember everything vibrates and is in motion, and the speed/rate at which it vibrates determines its consciousness. As I was learning to own my power as a Creator, I realized that my thoughts, words, reactions, feelings, actions, and beliefs affected the external reality that was showing up for me every day through my vibrational state. It is important to have patience and to love yourself, as it is not always easy to master this process. It is one thing to understand the complex relationship between our external reality and our inner mind; however, it is a completely different step to become proficient in directing and managing it.

The Law of Rhythm

The Law of Rhythm states that everything has its own unique timing or cycle. For example, the four seasons bring with them different weather patterns; the tides of the sea are in a constant ebb and flow; and in life, we all have a time to be born and a time to die. This helps us to be patient with our process because we each have our own divine timing. We tend to compare ourselves to others and judge ourselves as not being as far enough along in the process. However, there is no contest or competition in this evolution; we are all created equally and are allowed to set our own pace. We will all get there, step into our uniqueness, and become Creators of our reality. It is important to allow yourself the space to enjoy this process.

The Law of Alignment

This brings us to the Law of Alignment. We will become better at manifesting our reality as we master our Creator Matrix. Once we realize that we create our reality, we can practice consciously by observing and choosing which thought forms we allow, taking responsibility for our personal energetic field, and directing our energy toward what we will manifest. This is what alignment is all about: synchronizing the frequency and vibration within our Creator Matrix with what we wish to manifest. Remember, we must contain what we wish to manifest. If we have not cleared out our limiting beliefs and created a healthy physical environment from the cellular level up, we might not be able to contain or take responsibility for our desired creation. For example, I started my health coaching business despite never having gone to business school. This was tremendously overwhelming at first. I was not very good at managing my finances at the time and, as I've previously discussed, was constantly giving my energy away in all forms, including money. It took me years to even charge for my healing sessions. I was unable to contain the vision at first because my energy was not aligned to growth and success. If we want to stay small and have less responsibility, we will have a smaller container. If, on the other hand, we wish to have a large container, we must be willing to take the extra responsibility. Through my business, I have learned to balance and manage my finances and my energy, and I feel much happier in all areas of life.

The Law of Action

Change of any kind cannot happen without some form of movement. This brings us to the next law, which is the Law of Action. Many of my clients find it difficult to know when to act and when to refrain from acting; they jump into decisions too quickly, without listening to their "sixth sense" and inner wisdom, and then regret their choices later on. Others suffer from "analysis paralysis," where they have trouble making any decisions, and so miss out on opportunities that could have moved them toward their desired creations. As I learned to follow my intuition, I learned to trust my inner "knowing" and make better and more timely decisions. Remembering that there are no "right" or "wrong" choices, because we are here on Earth to experience anything and everything, helped me to apply this process without judgment and with more self-love.

The Law of Correspondence

The Law of Correspondence tells us that our physical world functions the same way as the etheric world. This law states, "As above, so below." As we master our Creator Matrix, we learn that energy and matter are the same and behave the same way. Matter is a denser form of energy. As we transition away from duality, this law will remain; however, the fabric of reality will have changed, and this will affect the base of how we function and interact.

The Law of Cause and Effect

This brings us to one of the most important laws, the Law of Cause and Effect. Through experiencing duality, we learn about cause and effect. In religious and spiritual terms, "We reap what we sow." Realizing that we create the effects of our behavior is a significant part of our evolution.

The Law of Compensation

The Law of Cause and Effect helps us to understand the Law of Compensation. We will be rewarded (or not) based on our behavior and actions. Some refer to this as karma. Transitioning out of duality will free us from our energetic distortions (karma) as we will rise above polarity and master our ability to manage all aspects of our reality as well as our Creator Matrix. Living multidimensionally, we will become the best, most actualized versions of ourselves, and will learn to receive abundance on all levels as we attract many positive blessings into our reality.

The Law of Perpetual Transmutation of Energy

The next law has to do with our ability to change. This law is called the Law of Perpetual Transmutation of Energy. We have free will on this planet—and, through our choices, we have the ability to change our state of being. So often, in the past, we believed that our environment (the people, places, or conditions surrounding us) needed to change in order for us to transform. This, however, is not how the Law of Perpetual

Transformation of Energy works. The higher frequencies have the ability to transform the lower frequencies. If we can hold a higher frequency, the world around us will shift its frequency to match ours and attract a corresponding world to us. Those of us who have learned to hold light and the higher frequencies to help the rest of the planet transform are often referred to as "lightworkers."

The Law of Relativity

We often compare our lives with those of others who seem to be in more ideal situations than we are. We can also feel compassion for others who are struggling. The Law of Relativity shows us how, in this physical world, we have learned through relationship and comparison, and this is why we have experienced duality. We learn about light through seeing darkness. We learn about cold by understanding heat. This law helps us accept all situations without judgment—to realize that everything is relative and in relationship to everything else, and that everyone is given a series of lessons to learn in their lives. There will always be those who appear "better off" or "worse off" than us. Detaching from the experience of duality helps us realize that we are not completely dependent on the story or experience we are having. We always have a choice about how to look at it. As we integrate, we will stop comparing ourselves and reside instead in the frequency of appreciation and gratitude for all differences.

The Law of Detachment

This brings us to the Law of Detachment, which is probably one of the most difficult laws to master. Being too attached to any outcome we wish to manifest stops the creative process. A master Creator lives in the "now" moment with complete trust in their manifestation. When we become attached, we feel that we need the outcome we are envisioning—that our happiness and fulfillment depends on it. In other words, we believe we need to control the process, which stops the flow of energy. Master Creators trust that intention and alignment alone will bring their creations to them.

I had to learn this lesson the hard way when I was experiencing fertility challenges while trying to conceive my second child. I wanted a second pregnancy as many of my friends and family were already on their third or fourth children. I became needy, obsessive, and attached to a pregnancy that had not yet manifested. I was living in the future. It wasn't until I let go of the need for the pregnancy, focused on my work, and gave the future over to my higher power that I managed to conceive. I literally gave it over to the universe, and I prayed to God. In order to create anything, we have to trust the process, live in the moment, and focus on what we can control right now, which is our internal state.

The Law of Polarity

The Law of Polarity looks specifically at dualistic opposition. Everything is equal and opposite and has two "poles"—for example, right and wrong, good and bad, up and down. In duality, there are two sides to everything. When people have a belief system or opinions that pertain to politics, education, environment, healthcare, etc., they own their belief system as though it is the only absolute truth. The Law of Polarity shows that there is always an equally valid opposite truth. When we get stuck in duality, we are unable to see the opposite as having any validity. We are seeing this challenge showing up between people and groups of people throughout the world at this time. As we pierce the illusion of duality and belief systems, we will begin to see both sides of the "poles." We can then rise above polarity and into a more integrated, holistic viewpoint.

The Law of Gender

While the Law of Polarity looks at opposition, the Law of Gender focuses on the duality of masculine and feminine (yang and yin). This law governs how, on the physical planet, we have manifested life itself. The energy of the masculine is giving, and the feminine is receiving. This is illustrated in the way we reproduce with an egg and sperm. Both of these energies need to be present within us and in our creative cycle in order for us to manifest optimally.

When we transcend duality, each Creator will have integrated the "male" and "female" (yang and yin) aspects of themselves and will no longer need to look outside of themselves to find balance and fulfillment. It's even possible that, in the future, we will be able to manifest children through thought alone!

The Law of Allowing

We looked at the Law of Allowing in Chapter Two. This law has helped both me and my clients to take responsibility for what we have created and what we want to create. Personally, I learned to become conscious of what I was allowing in my life (certain relationships, food, jobs, social media, etc.), and how I was reacting to it. I learned to flow with what was showing up and trust that I could manage these challenges. I got in the habit of taking a breath before reacting to anything. This Law of Allowing helped me expand my possibilities and grow my container to allow more expansive thoughts and outcomes. I learned to use empowering words rather than disempowering words, and ask, "What if this seemingly impossible thing *is* possible?" In this way, the Law of Allowing has given me the courage to live my life to the fullest.

***

As we wake up to how our world operates, we understand that "structure is function" on every level of body, mind, and spirit, and that the structures we build and maintain within our Creator Matrix determine our experience of the world around us. When we become conscious of the Universal Laws and how they work, we can begin to step into our full power as Creators. Instead of resisting the flow of the universe, we will learn to work with it, and let it carry us.

Becoming Quantum: Looking at Densities

Harnessing the power of your Creator Matrix requires integrating all aspects of yourself. When you do this, you will own your Creatorship and consciously make choices that condense timelines. As you, as a Creator, take more responsibility for co-creating your experiences with Universal Source, your environment, your cells, and your body, you will be given various opportunities to refine your skills and approach life from a quantum perspective. If your Creator Matrix is not integrated, different aspects of yourself will remain disconnected, creating energetic blockages and slowing your creative process. As you integrate, you will become whole, healed, and able to show up authentically.

As the quantum world reveals itself to us, we will start to rely more on our psychic senses to recognize, consciously interact with, and heal ourselves at four different levels of existence: physical, mental, emotional, and spiritual. As we do this, our frequency will rise, and our self-love and self-empowerment will be restored. From this experience of healing, we will begin to live with the knowingness that we exist multidimensionally. Our ability to sense will increase, and we will begin sensing multidimensionally. Through this process we will become master Creators.

I call this state "quantum living."

Everything that we see, and everything that we don't see, in both the materialistic and non-materialistic realms, vibrates at different speeds/rates on a scale. A "density" is a specific scale or range within which energy and/or consciousness is vibrating. Matter will express itself differently depending on the different densities it exists in. On a physical level, the density of matter is expressed as different states of solid, liquid, and gas. Spiritually, each density will hold completely different phases of evolutionary lessons and experiences. The transition from one density to the next is the ascension process. On Earth, we are currently experiencing an ascension from the third density to the fourth density, and ultimately to the fifth density. This is exciting! We can compare this to the transition we make from lower school to higher school education. Each level provides different lessons and experiences; and as we advance, each experience gives us greater independence and autonomy.

What differentiates each density is the level of light it contains. As we evolve, we are increasing the amount of light we can hold in our physical bodies. In other words, our bodies are becoming less dense or solid. In this transition, we are reaching progressively lighter states of being.

If we look back at our discussion about science and light, we remember that the more light we hold, the higher the frequency (speed of vibration) of the photons within our field. Lorie Ladd, in her recent book *The Divine Design*, writes, "Physical evolution occurs when a form in the Earth's Plane begins to physically anchor into the next highest dimensional field. The form is holding the frequencies of that field, and that field becomes their new reality. This can only occur when Earth is holding more light in her form, increasing her frequency, while simultaneously clearing out the density or lower frequency light from within her form."[2] She continues on to explain that densities are created from the human collective consciousness. As our human consciousness expands, more light and information will be available for each person to access.

Contemplating the impact of different densities on our health and life experience, I was humbled by the fact that we do not know and understand everything at this time. Below is a table explaining the possible densities of our evolutionary path. If we look at this from a higher viewpoint, of course, there is no separation; in fact, these densities have always coexisted. However, as we transcend densities, what we see, perceive, and experience will change in relation to the amount of light we carry and our own individual consciousness. As we make more connections and begin to hold more light, our physical bodies will lighten as well. Some refer to this as the change from a *homo sapiens* to a "homo-luminous" being.

As we transform our own energy into a higher, less dense reality, our perceptions will change, and we will become more efficient at reading energy and using it. Densities exist in the mind of the one who observes them; if our consciousness only allows us to see everything in parts, then seeing something as a whole is not possible. In order to make the shift to higher densities, we need to transcend the old belief systems, thought patterns, fears, and emotions by releasing them and replacing them with new ones that serve our present consciousness in a better way.

The Law of One, which we explored earlier in this chapter, was channeled by a group that exists in the Sixth Density and call themselves Ra. This information was channeled through a medium named Carla Rueckert. Ra claims that there are seven densities of experience in a universe and that other universes also exist. Once a soul completes its evolution through the seventh density, it graduates to the next seven densities in another universe. There are lessons that need to be mastered in each density, and the process continues. There is no ending; life is eternal, just as we are eternal.[3]

According to Ra, the first density in our universe is the experience of "being." The evolution of elementals, rocks, minerals, and water exist in this density. The second density is about experiencing growth and movement and involves the evolution of DNA and the plant and animal kingdoms. The third density is focused on learning about the consciousness of "self" and is the first density where humans have existed. Here, we experience duality and much suffering in our storylines. Due to this fact, we have the shortest lifetimes. In this density we must learn how to maneuver and choose how we will react to the dualistic stories we experience.

As mentioned above, the "awakening" for many of us at this time is about transitioning from the third to the fourth density. Here, we are learning how to be in authentic service to others, to be in our hearts, and to genuinely love ourselves and all of humanity. The fifth density happens when we as humans have completely integrated our Creator Matrix. In that density, we have gained access to all "knowingness" and can easily connect to quantum fields of information. In the fifth density, manifestation is instant. Our heavy, dense bodies will have transitioned from a carbon base to a crystalline structure.

From the sixth density onward, our lessons are about unity consciousness, which is a combination of mastering unconditional love and wisdom. Here we are mastering service to Source as we are becoming more aligned and connected to the Prime Creator. We can exist as individual beings and/or groups of beings and can guide the creative process of this universe as a whole. Many spiritual masters have channeled about the experiences within other more advanced densities. However, after a certain point we are unable to perceive all the lessons and experiences that each of these will provide, as they are so far from our current level of understanding and awareness.

As we evolve toward higher consciousness with a more developed light body, we will become more whole. In the heavy, third-density energy, we feel things more slowly, separately, and chaotically. By experiencing this separation, we can now appreciate connecting to the whole in a more conscious way. If we are energy, science is showing us that quantum frequency is the only difference between us as individuals, and the only thing standing between us and ascension into the higher densities.

Some of the concepts presented in this chapter may be challenging. You may even be learning of them for the first time. You may be looking for facts that will provide absolute proof that densities exist, and that the Universal Laws are in fact at play in your life.

Throughout history, visionaries and scientists have explored ideas and concepts before they could prove them scientifically. This reach into the unknown is the basis of discovery. As you read this chapter, I encourage you to feel how these ideas resonate with you at a "sixth sense" or "knowingness" level, and how they bring understanding to the experiences you might be having. Perhaps this will provide comfort and provide some explanation for the mysteries that life has presented to you. Or it will simply leave you with more questions. As we have already discussed in this book, science is beginning to challenge some of the ways we perceive our reality. For me personally, understanding Universal Laws, densities, and dimensions has brought clarity to my experience and expanded my awareness.

DENSITY	WHO/WHERE	MAIN FOCUS
1st	Elemental level: Rocks, minerals, water	Base of creation and being
2nd	DNA, plants, lower animal kingdom	Unique consciousness of biology, growing from being to movement
3rd	Human beings	Duality, illusion of separation Consciousness continues to grow toward self-reflection Service to self Self-love and self-worth
4th	Human beings	Observation Self-reflection Awareness of the subconscious Moving toward heart-based living and unity consciousness Recognition that we are Creators
5th	Human beings (light, crystalline bodies), Ascended masters	Coherent heart consciousness Complete experience of unity consciousness Being in/condensing multiple timelines Service to others and Source Integrated Creator Matrix Instant manifestation
6th	Ascended masters Group conscious beings Etheric light wave forms Sacred geometry Multiverses (beyond our universe) Integrated Source consciousness	Non-physical existence Wisdom and unity consciousness All-knowingness and ideas of creation Creation of worlds, cosmoses, galaxies God consciousness Unconditional love Infinity

Carl Sagan Explains Dimensions

Many people refer to dimensions as "otherworldly." The word "dimensions" has many meanings, but in terms of understanding our reality it can refer to a measurement of something in our physical space and/or different planes of existence.

The word "dimension" is often used interchangeably with the word "density" when discussing our evolutionary leap in consciousness at this time, however there are slight but important differences. Whereas "density" refers to the amount of light that can be contained within a certain body, "dimension" refers to a perspective of the universe: what we can see and what bandwidth of information we are able to perceive. In other words, a field of possibilities.

People living within a specific dimension can only see what is in their range of perception. When we hear the word "dimension," we tend to think of it as a destination, a place separate from this place that we can go to or connect with. However, science is showing us that this is not the case. A dimension pertains to a particular space or field that we exist in and that gives us unique possibilities to experience.

Carl Sagan was an astronomer and planetary scientist who questioned everything. He once said: "Science is more than a body of knowledge; it is a way of thinking." In the 1980s, he wrote a book entitled *Cosmos,* and hosted a television series that explored who we are and our relationship to the cosmos. Back then, Sagan was already discussing the concept of fourth-dimension reality, as if he was already preparing us for the shift we are now experiencing. Specifically, he described our inability to understand multiple dimensions from our limited dimensional perspective.

In a YouTube video entitled "Cosmos-Carl Sagan-4th Dimension," he describes different dimensions that allow us different perspectives.[4] He begins by comparing our reality to that of Flatland—a place where everyone and everything is completely flat and can perceive the world through width and length, but not height. Similarly, these Flatland dwellers understand going forward and backward, but not up or down.

The Flatlander cannot perceive three-dimensional reality; they can only perceive back/forth and left/right, but not up/down. They have no context for it, and no experience of it, since that up/down reality is not part of their current dimension.

Our universe has many levels that are evolving toward more advanced and complicated dimensional realities. At this moment we are running into the same limited understanding as the Flatland population. However, as we grow in consciousness, we will move beyond the three-dimensional reality of up/down, back/forth, right/left; in fact, as we move into the fourth-dimensional reality, we will be able to perceive right angles to up/down, back/forth, and right/left. Fourth-dimensional awareness will expand our ability to perceive the complexity of our universe. As we transition to this higher dimension, we will gain more freedom of movement, abilities, and possibilities. As the higher density brings more light into matter, the higher dimension will mirror this change and the template of existence will allow for more movement within space and time. When we shift to a new dimension, our physical length, width, depth, and space/time parameters will become expanded.

To make the difference between density and dimension more clear: the first three densities all exist in the same dimension. All aspects of these densities have access on some level to up/down, back/forth, and right/left. Now, as this great shift unfolds, we are changing our space and time limitations. The rules that governed the third density are evolving; we are now transitioning to be able to perceive right angles to up/down back/forth right/left. We are in a quantum jump of awareness and shift in what we can perceive in our reality. The multidimensional template or field we inhabit is changing. We can compare this to a new playground that will allow us new equipment (technologies) to develop new abilities and expanded experiences. We will transcend the limitations of the third dimension as we awaken to see more and know more. Our life lessons, storylines, and experiences will also change as they mirror this new dimensional reality.

Living in a multidimensional world will require us to expand our perception, awareness, and consciousness. Each person will need to do this in their own time, and in their own way. Imagine what more we will see, learn, and understand as we continue to transition to this amazing higher dimension of possibilities.

The First Five Densities

FIRST DENSITY

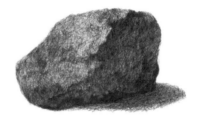

When I was at Georgetown University, I took a theology class that really impacted my idea of consciousness. The priest, our instructor, taught us about a theologian named Pierre Teilhard de Chardin. Teilhard was a Jesuit philosopher and paleontologist. Born in France in 1881, he loved nature, rocks, and stones in particular. He believed that consciousness existed on all levels and densities and looked to science to understand our spiritual evolution. He literally believed that rocks had consciousness. Teilhard had tremendous powers of observation and spoke about atoms having some sort of "love bonding." This first density is therefore the simplest form of consciousness in our universe.

At that time in my life, this was revolutionary information for me. This first dimension of existence is the densest in the physical form. It is the elemental level and the basis of creation. From my perspective, rocks and stones always appeared solid. To learn that there was more space than matter in them, and that the atoms within them were constantly in motion, was a mind-blowing thought. Teilhard wrote many books trying to show that mankind is evolving mentally and socially toward a unity consciousness. He wanted to look at science for answers about human evolution. Today, as we are learning more about metaphysics and quantum science, the connections between science and spirituality are becoming increasingly clear, and many consider Teilhard to be a pioneer in this field.[5][6]

SECOND DENSITY

The second density involves the lower animal kingdom, vegetables, plants, and trees. When I was young, I was very fearful of wild animals and never wanted to be alone in nature, particularly at night. This separated me from nature. As I was awakening, I became more conscious and connected to this second density. I could feel the frequency and purity of it. I always loved my pets (dogs, cats, fish, and birds), and I was fascinated by the differences between them and their unconditional love for humanity. Eventually, I began to connect more to plant life, and I felt more aligned and grounded in nature.

Second density is about the development of organic physical matter. It is about the development of DNA; and as there is progression through this stage, there is growth toward independence. Therefore, if this stage starts with the consciousness of a tree, it ends with the consciousness of an animal. Animals, like us, are growing in their ability to move and connect to their environment through their biology. They are evolving toward having an identity and experiencing self and will.

Several years ago, as I walked outside, the willow tree in my garden suddenly seemed to communicate with me that it was in serious trouble. Out of curiosity, I called my gardener. He said that the tree was indeed rotting from the inside out and that I should have it cut down immediately. I could not accept this because the tree was still so beautiful. So, I asked for a second opinion from a tree surgeon in our area. The tree surgeon said that he could heal the tree with medicine and a pruning of the branches, and he did exactly that. Now the willow stands stronger than ever. I continue to feel a deep connection of joy with this tree.

As we learn to connect to different densities, we understand how to communicate with all that is existing within each density. By doing so, we will create greater harmony throughout the multiverse.

THIRD DENSITY

The third is the density we as humans have lived in for eons. It has the most dense and heavy energies that humans can experience. Third-density energy is very slow. The largest attribute of this density is that humans are in a survival-based, competitive, and dualistic matrix. We can get stuck in our storylines, the intense feelings that can come up in them, and experience those feelings as suffering. In this density, people do not yet realize that they are creating their own reality. They experience their stories in a linear manner and in opposition by playing different roles, such as victim, perpetrator, or savior. Furthermore, some can become trapped in life stories where an issue such as "lack" or "strife" is the central theme. In such a case, the duality being played out is between lack and abundance. An example of this would be constantly believing that you cannot create abundance yourself, but that it must come from something outside of yourself, like your partner, the government, or another organization. Similarly, you may have two homes from which to choose, but purchase the less expensive one as you don't believe that you are capable of keeping up with the mortgage payments and other responsibilities associated with owning a larger house.

In this third-density reality, we have needed to learn who we are in relation to others. We have learned about our ego, and asked, "Who am I?" In my healing work, I have noticed that the first three chakras correspond to the first three densities. In order to transition out of the third density, each of us must heal these first three chakras. We must learn to create safety on all levels (body, mind, and spirit), connect to our creative spark, realize that we have a Creator Matrix and are the Creator—and, as a result, feel and know our connection to everything. When we heal the first three chakras, our need to prove our worthiness and importance will vanish as we will understand that we are all that is; we are the great "I am." When this happens, the only limitation in manifesting will be what thoughts we allow.

When we want to create something in third-density energy, we do so from a linear perspective. Let's say that you want to buy a new house. You imagine the house in great detail: how many bedrooms, the layout of the kitchen, and even that porch swing you've always dreamed about. Then, almost immediately, your mind is brought back to your present financial reality. You think, "If I want this house, I'll need to get a promotion." However, the next week, you lose your job. Feeling defeated, you give up on your idea of a new house because your mind is solely concerned with survival issues. The vision of your dream house evaporates because your mind is obsessed with the thought, "I need to get a job fast." If we create from our thoughts, linear thinking has already limited our possibilities. By thinking something is not possible, we make it impossible. This is how most of us have been living and existing in our current reality, with the illusion that our fate is dictated by a force outside of ourselves. It's a rare person who can hold the vision of their dream home in third-density energy for long enough to manifest it. Instead, most people think thoughts with many conditions based on their programming and limiting beliefs. The moment the dream home comes up, the next thought is always about the "how"—that they have to work harder, have to win the lottery, or wait until someone dies in order to inherit their money. There is no room for possibilities heretofore unheard-of or unexperienced.

In the third density, most of us live our lives from a purely physical standpoint and are unable to see beyond the physical matrix our senses can perceive. We can experience life as feeling separate from all that is. We can feel separate from each other, separate from our physical reality, and separate from all dimensions of existence. In this density, our sciences and arts have progressed only as far as our physical understanding. Many of us search for happiness through our accomplishments and acquiring something outside of ourselves—from basic physical needs like food, shelter, comfort, and sex, to power and social status, to luxury material goods.

Through our life stories, we have been learning to master the materialistic world. Now, it is time for us to transcend the material and look beyond the purely physical experience. In the third density, we learn to see through the illusion of matter, and to rise above duality and the pain and suffering it brings to our life stories. The true pain in these stories is, of course, the separation they cause us to feel. In a sense, therefore, the real lesson we are learning is that there is no separation, and that we are connected to everything and everyone. Through connecting to everything and everyone, we become healed and enlightened.

As I listened to many of my clients' stories, certain life themes with fears and emotional blockages are continually carried on throughout their lives until complete healing ensues. Whether it is drama around relationships, money, health, career, loss or basic survival, our stories will repeat because they are imbalanced, and this imbalanced energy seeks resolution. For example, as I shared before, when I was younger, I began to observe a pattern of thinking that had an immediate effect on my life. I had frequent experiences surrounding people dying from illness, car accidents, or suicide. Consequently, I became preoccupied with a tremendous mistrust in the health of my body and noticed therefore that my body would feel even more vulnerable to illness, disease, or accidents. Just how the concept goes, the more I focused on ill health and accidents, the more I attracted this very thing into my life and body. I would tell my parents that I had a stomachache, and they would take me to the doctor. As soon as the doctor said there was nothing to worry about, I began to feel better immediately. It was a spontaneous recovery! As mentioned in the earlier part of the book, I became more aware of this pattern through working with José, the kinesiologist, and other healers as I got older. They helped me to further heal the preoccupation and mistrust that I had of my body and the environment. José found that I carried with me, on a deeply subconscious level, a fear that I was unhealthy, and that I had an inherent mistrust of my body and the outside world. Through reprogramming my subconscious, I was able to release these deep-seated fears, and, with critical observation,

I can now catch myself when this old thought pattern resurfaces. The difference now is that the thoughts carry no emotional fear when they do return. The lesson for me, therefore, was to learn to trust that my body was healthy, and my environment is safe for me to maneuver in. I have learned that even if my body feels sick, it will rebalance itself and become well again. I have also learned to be more grounded and pay more attention to my environment. By creating a feeling of safety, I have had fewer accidents. However, we can all have different themes that resurface or need attention.

The place where we most deeply experience separation in the third density is in our relationships. Our subconscious can have a tremendous impact on our relationship fears and patterns. Dependence and independence within relationships are common themes. José once said to me, "A healthy relationship is one where both parties are completely independent and enjoy and encourage watching the other grow and blossom." This goes for family and friend relationships as well as intimate partnerships. I have learned that the feeling of "needing" someone else to fulfill you may lead to an unhealthy attachment. When we desperately "need" someone or something, we are giving our power away to that person or thing, instead of owning our own power as a Creator.

The second major issue in relationships is often communication. How do we communicate through our thoughts and feelings? We all have different opinions, personalities, ways of coping with conflict, different needs for power and control, subconscious fears, and strengths and weaknesses. Most importantly, we all have different levels of conscious awareness. All of these affect how we react to, interact with, and ultimately co-create with those around us.

As we learn that we create our own reality alongside others, two issues will be mastered. The first is learning to trust ourselves and accept our differences. The second is learning to navigate our challenges with a more holistic perspective. Compassion and acceptance will help us to grow, move forward, and connect to ourselves and others, which is what love—the nature of the universe—is all about. As we become more self-aware in the third density, we are experiencing what love is, how to give it, how to receive it, how to feel it, how to heal it, and how to connect with it.

FOURTH DENSITY

As we transition to the fourth density, we rise above duality. We learn that we are connected to all that is. The veil between our physical reality and other dimensions becomes thinner. We gain greater access to our Akashic Records and begin to experience memories and remembrances (like healing past lives and unresolved issues) that can make us feel that we are living in an unreal world. Once we understand what is happening, we can gain compassion for what we have been through, and the pain and trauma in our Creator Matrix can be healed. When we do this, our bodies will literally "lighten up."

In order to offload the heavier energy of the third density, we must go through a process of self-observation and self-awareness. At first, this process focuses on the "self" and self-healing, but as we gain more light and perspective, the focus will shift to the "other." Meaningful connections are only possible when we can love ourselves and others without conditions. This requires that we live more from our hearts—but we can only live in our hearts once we have healed the wounds of our hearts. By doing so, we can transcend the duality of right/wrong and dark/light. We can observe our thoughts, emotions, people, and storylines. Are they based on fear, or based on love? Once we can forgive and let go of these wounds, we can reside in this space without blockages.

One of the fears I had to overcome was a fear of rejection. If I wanted to step into my power and carry this light, I would need to heal my heart from the wounds of humiliation I had suffered in my past for thinking differently than others. It can sometimes feel easier to stick with the frequency of the crowd and not admit that we think differently than others, as a sense of belonging is particularly important for many of us. Being different can threaten this feeling of safety and connection. However, I now feel far more accepting of myself than I used to and have let go of needing to please everyone around me. I have less anxiety when others disagree with me, and more acceptance of my reactions; instead of retreating and hiding, I have learned to love myself even more in these situations. Once we realize the power of living from a heart/love-based reality, we can let go of our addiction to dramatic, dualistic stories and instead choose stories that bring us more fulfillment and self-actualization.

One of my spiritual teachers once said to me, "Always stay attractive." I reflected on what this meant for me and realized that one quality all truly attractive people share is self-love. As I grow in consciousness, I realize that there is always a choice in how to handle a conflict. Handling the conflict as the best version of myself means acting from a state of compassion and love for myself and others.

Making this transition from third to fourth-density reality is usually a gradual process. Old habits and patterns will resurface until they are completely cleared. I began truly awakening around the year 2000 and, as I have already shared, I had to heal a great deal of my ancestral female line. Releasing ancestral family karma and outdated belief systems has taken time, but it has been worth the wait. I believe that this process can now go much faster for many people, as the energy is much lighter and there is more information available. However, in the transition period, many can still fall back into patterns of victimhood and powerlessness. Personal growth and change are the name of the game.

So, what does it mean to rise into fourth-density reality and live from our hearts? This is a good question. I believe that if we interviewed 1,000 people, we would invariably receive 1,000 different opinions. However, certain themes overlap. Heart awareness is a deep feeling of self-connection that can bring us in touch with our inner power and innate knowingness. With this connection to our knowingness, we can become more true to ourselves and authentic in our choices and behaviors. We can receive messages from Universal Source/ the quantum field, and consequently feel happier and more balanced. Remember, the heart has the largest electromagnetic field in the body, and is like an enormous walk-in library with a possible connection to all that is. When we are connected to the electromagnetic field, we are "plugged in," and we must be connected to this field to fully benefit from its power. The greater our connection, the greater our access to this lighter-density energy, and the more we will be able to see greater possibilities for our own lives and those of others.

Many of us are becoming aware of narcissism as a negative personality trait that can be dominant in unhealthy, painful relationships. Like all psychiatric disorders, it can be rooted from trauma and disconnection. If we look at narcissism with third-density glasses, then we will view narcissists as the "bad guys," the perpetrators. However, as we transition to the fourth density, we will find a higher perspective and develop compassion for all the players in the story.

Instead of looking at this as a condition, we can see it as a stage in our development to learn about ourselves and our own personal power. The "service of self" or "living from the ego" is a natural stage of development in being able to reach an authentic level of service toward others and mankind. It is important to understand that "service to self" is an integral part of learning how to love and care for oneself. Some of us learn from playing the roles of "pleasers" and "givers", while others will inhabit the role of the "takers." The energy of both relies on what they give or get from the outside world, instead of realizing that they have the power within them to generate whatever they need or desire at any time. This can be compared to a well. If your well is empty, you constantly need to work in order to fill it. If you learn how to fill your well, you can more easily give water to others. As we evolve, this state of replenishing our energy fields with love and light will be instantaneous; we will want and need for nothing as we will be abundant on all levels.

It is necessary to love oneself completely to truly serve mankind; and as people are growing in consciousness, they are learning to love themselves completely. As mentioned before, I have learned to care for and love myself completely by practicing deep breathing, meditation, yoga, prayer, and other practices daily. When I do these practices regularly, I am better able to access higher-frequency emotions and gain greater access to multidimensional living.

In the fourth-density reality, we will become more integrated with our Creator Matrix. We will also begin to use our imagination more, and experience our imagined reality as being "real." We will begin to play more easily with the energy of the quantum field, and the "mystical" and "impossible" will become possible as we increase our perception. As this is happening, we may experience physical symptoms such as dizziness. Our dreams may seem more real, and our reality more dream-like. We will begin to use our creative abilities on all levels of existence. On a physical level, we can paint, sing, build, or write—however, on other levels, we will begin to create through new techniques that integrate all aspects of body, mind, and spirit. These may include creating new quantum financial systems, new artistic ways of quantum expression, and new ways of quantum healing. Living multidimensionally can seem almost unreal at times, and this ascension will indeed shift our perception of reality.

We will also evolve how we deal with emotions. Emotional intelligence is also about turning negative emotions into positive emotions and realizing that we have a choice concerning which emotional states we want to "hang out" in. As we get accustomed to living in higher emotional frequencies like joy, love, gratitude, and peace, we will attract people and situations into our lives that mimic those emotional frequencies. We will be freer to speak our authentic truths without judgment. This will have a ripple effect throughout the world. As more and more people shift into this heart-based reality, we will transition into a collective connectedness that is based on love. "I" will become "we" as we harmonize together. When my students lament that they cannot help all of the people suffering in the world, I always respond by explaining the ripple effect. When you change your frequency, you change the world.

When a critical mass of humanity shifts into fourth-density living, the entire nature of our lived reality will change. Moreover, we will be poised on the brink of our next phase of ascension—the shift into fifth-density reality.

FIFTH DENSITY

In earlier chapters, we looked at how consciousness affects energy. In her book, *Unlocking the Ancient Secrets to Healing*, Gail Lynn states, "Physical light behaves like a particle when we place our direct attention on it and as a wave when it is not being observed. This really gives us a lot of power to create our own reality." Where we direct our conscious attention will impact what we manifest—from the etheric to the physical. It takes practice to become comfortable and confident enough to manifest in this way. As we move into higher-density living, we can connect to a quantum field that is outside of this dualistic, heavier energy. In the past, when we played out the paradigm of duality, our essence has been split between the light and the dark as they were separated. To look at it another way, we will let go of "negative" as the dualistic opposite of "positive." Both the light/dark and negative/positive will become integrated into "one," and this will bring us to a completely new level of awareness.

By the time we have entered fifth-density reality, which is a state of being rather than a time or place, we will be in full command of our Creatorship. We will simply know that we create our reality and, as a result, will be in greater control of how we react to our outside world. We will choose and learn to inhabit the high-frequency states of joy and love. As we practice creating our reality on a daily basis and the energy within us becomes more crystalline, so too will our abilities increase and expand, allowing us more control over both our energy fields and our environment.

We will communicate via our psychic abilities and practice great control over our thought forms. We will be able to read others' energy and use healthy boundaries when interacting with others. There will be no more secrets; lying and deceiving others will no longer be possible or necessary.

So far in our reality, we have played out our stories between the dualistic energies of dark and light. Conflict and war, therefore, have been the norm as these energies have been in opposition. In the future, we will no longer need to fight wars as we will have integrated this polarity. Our illusion of separation will be over. We will realize that all of our thoughts, actions, and emotions impact the whole, and choose accordingly. This is the culmination of our shift from service of self to service of others that began in the third and fourth densities. In fifth-density reality, service of self and service of others are interconnected and directly affect each other in the now moment.

We will gain more responsibility and freedom and gladly accept it. With greater responsibility will come greater knowledge and abilities. In our current third-density reality, manifesting seems to take a great deal of effort, yet as we move into this higher fifth density we will manifest instantly and move matter with our thoughts. Imagine desiring a kale salad for dinner and having it appear on your table. Perhaps, at this point, eating will be more of a choice and not a necessity. Imagine that you'd like to present yourself twenty pounds thinner and with red hair, and then watch yourself transform in the mirror. Imagine living in Germany but wanting to be in Australia, and then appearing there with a thought. Some people think this cannot happen; others want this reality now. However, humanity is not prepared for this ability. It would be like giving a two-year-old the keys to a car. Until we can control our thought forms and become consciously aligned with our desires and *only* our desires, we will not gain this ability. As we grow and evolve, manifesting will become easier because we will know who we are—that we are truly magnificent, divine, and connected to Source energy.

In order to learn this skill, we also need to recognize our self-sabotaging habits that keep us from reaching our true potential as human beings. Learning to accept our greatness is part of the difficulty on Earth. For many people it can be hard to take responsibility for their reality or change the programs that have kept them small. Staying small and hiding can be far easier. Imagine a world where we all took full responsibility for ourselves, the world, and each other. Life would naturally then be more expansive, possibly offering more connections and mystical experiences. People would no longer feel a need to have power over one another, as they would understand the uselessness of that. People would be less concerned with getting revenge as they would realize that, because we are all connected, they would only be hurting themselves. Furthermore, the duality of arguing who is "right" and who is "wrong" will fade as more people realize that most opinions are based on belief systems and judgments, not absolutes. Our heart growth will help us transcend rigid beliefs and develop compassion for each other.

In third-density reality, we have had to work hard at staying in balance because we have been managing dualities. As we transcend this dualistic state, it will no longer be necessary to keep balance as the tension between the poles will no longer exist. Without imbalance, there will be no disease. As we will exist in high-frequency light, we will know how to care for ourselves and heal instantly. Our environment will no longer have a propensity toward illness, pain, or suffering. In the past, pain has helped to protect us and navigate our journey toward growth; there was a purpose to our suffering. In fifth-density reality, that will be a thing of the past; instead, we will trust that whatever emerges is for our ultimate good.

Trust also has a frequency. We need to consciously choose it. When we trust ourselves, we are this high frequency, and this will affect what we manifest.

As we learn that we can create abundance, we will be able to transmute any areas in ourselves that bring up "lack." We will no longer need to be vengeful, controlling, fearful, or selfish. In third-density reality, when we faced a conflict, we often would use defense mechanisms to protect ourselves from the unsafe feeling that was created. The defense mechanisms served us, as we lived in a world where everyone felt separate from one another. We have all used defense mechanisms as a way of protecting our fragile souls.

One of the more common defense mechanisms is denial. When the stories we create make us feel too vulnerable, we often deny what is happening as a way to avoid facing the truth.

For example, a business partner finds out that his co-partner has been embezzling money from the company without him knowing it. This situation causes the business partner to deny this reality as he is afraid to confront his co-partner. In a fifth-density world, the co-worker could not hide his cheating as everything becomes transparent. Nor would it be necessary to cheat as the co-partner would be an abundant Creator and would realize that cheating his partner hurts both him and the whole of the organization.

Another example is the defense mechanism known as projection. Projection is when we see and judge something in another person that we have not yet accepted and integrated within ourselves. Because of this imbalance, a person can become conscious of, disturbed by, and preoccupied with the (usually challenging) qualities of someone else, when they have exactly the same shadow qualities within themselves. Often, this mirroring can make them feel uncomfortable, so they decide that they do not like the other person. In fifth-density reality, our darkness, shadow sides, and unconscious will be integrated and therefore accepted. We will see things from a higher perspective and be aware of all connections. This will help us develop a tremendous compassion for each other, and we will be able to cherish the differences between us.

The New Twelve-Chakra System

As we upgrade our individual systems and make more connections to our Creator Matrix, we are awakening to a larger, more holistic chakra system. Until now, we have been aware of and had access to the seven chakras, which are where we physically connect to Source energy. As you will remember from Chapter Two, these correspond to the visible colors of the rainbow. As we grow in our abilities and connect to larger fields of light and information, our chakra system will change and expand. The new chakras will connect to higher-frequency, effervescent colors of gold and platinum.

Our whole mind, body, and spirit complex, which I have called our Creator Matrix, has also been called our *Merkabah*. The word, pronounced mer-ka-ba, comes from ancient Egypt and means "special field of light" (mer), "human spirit" (ka) and "body" (ba). In Hebrew the word means "chariot" or "cart." The Merkabah that encompasses our body, mind, and spirit/soul matrix has two tetrahedrons spinning in opposite directions that, together, connect us to Source energy.

The twelve-chakra system, unlike the seven-chakra system, extends far beyond the physical body. While the seven-chakra system starts at the crown of your head and ends at the base of your spine, the twelve-chakra system will extend from above your head to below your feet and into the Earth.

As we activate and open our heart chakra, we will naturally connect to these other chakras both above and below our bodies. Once we start to connect to our higher self, we will activate the Soul Star, which is located about six inches above the crown chakra. This will bring us in touch with higher guidance from the Universal Field and start our acceleration into more multidimensional living. We will also discover the Earth Star chakra, located about twelve inches below the soles of our feet, and which connects us to Earth's magnetic-crystalline grid. When we connect to the Earth Star, we can access and connect our energy to Earth's magnetic core, which helps us stabilize our body's energetic system. As we ascend, it becomes more and more important to learn how to ground our light with the energies of Mother Earth as this brings us stability, health, and strength.

As we further expand our awareness, we will connect to our Galactic Gateway, which is about three feet above our head. This will connect us with our galactic mission—or, in more practical terms, our reason for incarnation in this life. Both the Soul Star and the Galactic Gateway help us transcend time and space as we know it, and we begin to live multidimensionally. As we continue to ascend, we can activate the upper gateways, the Universal Gateway and the Cosmic Gateway, which will connect us to the angelic realms and higher light beings. As more of our dormant DNA is energized, we will stimulate these chakras, and create a stronger, more activated Merkabah.

While all of this may feel very far-fetched or distant, it truly is not. Our first step in evolving into twelve-chakra, fifth-density beings is to become conscious of the possibilities. Step two is to learn to clean, protect, and connect to both Earth energy and higher-dimensional energies daily. Step three is learning to activate and strengthen our entire Merkabah. Once the first steps are taken toward accessing this level of our Creatorship, the rest will naturally follow.

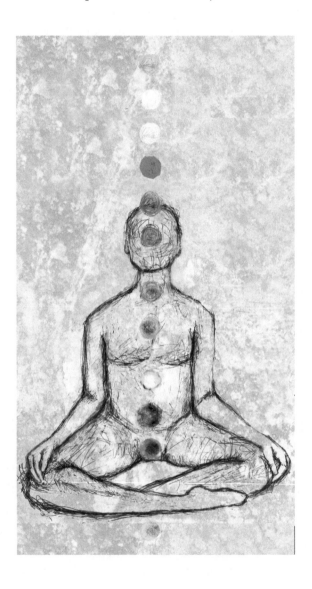

Making the Shift

The very energy that we play with every day is changing. As a collective, we are beginning to tap into far more expansional energies—the energies of the fourth and fifth densities. Where until now we have only been able to access linear, third-density energies, this change in our ability to access and use energy that is lighter, less dense, and more multidimensional will feel magical.

We will be able to access a grid of information about everyone and everything, on our own and without the need for a computer. We will develop and refine our higher intuitive (sixth sense) abilities. As our perception grows, so too will our ability to master our energy and energetic field. We will eventually develop abilities such as telekinesis and psychokinesis (the ability to move physical objects with our thoughts), as well as remote viewing skills that will allow us to see and know exactly what is going on anywhere on Earth. Furthermore, we may even be able to see what is happening throughout our galaxy and other universes and travel there instantly.

Over the last twenty years, I have been connecting more and more to these intuitive aspects in myself. As a child, I was afraid of them. For instance, when my third-grade teacher committed suicide, I could feel her around me but didn't know how to put that feeling into words or share it with others. As a nurse, I became aware that I could feel others' emotions, and this led me to a knowingness about what they were thinking. When I awakened to my healing abilities, I could immediately feel energies, frequencies, and densities; when I was working in somebody else's aura, I could receive information about that person. Later on, I could simply think about someone and connect to their Akash or what I call their "grid." When I started coaching people and helping them heal themselves, I often used this ability. I also had a knowingness for myself of what to do in the now for my future, and what direction to take and not to take. This ability to transcend the limiting five senses is the beginning of multidimensional living. The impending Age of Information or Age of Aquarius will indeed bring us from third-density to fifth-density existence. We will live in our hearts and be connected to the frequency of love. The love frequency also brings us into the frequency of being conscious Creators because our bodies will hold more light, and light is information. We will be more connected to all that is, and the illusion of separation will fade.

Chapter Summary

- The twelve fundamental Universal Laws of Consciousness help us transition into multidimensional living.

- Living multidimensionally allows us to experience reality beyond the matrix of our physical form. This quantum reality is becoming our new reality, and our ability to think multidimensionally is our entry point into this quantum existence or quantum living.

- With the knowingness that we exist multidimensionally, our ability to sense will increase; we will rely more on our psychic senses and begin sensing multidimensionally. Our frequency will rise, our self-love and self-empowerment will be restored, and we will become master Creators.

- We are currently experiencing an ascension from third density to fourth density in a transition to fifth density. As we evolve, we are increasing the amount of light we can hold in our physical bodies and our bodies are becoming less dense or solid.

- Where "density" refers to the amount of light that can be contained within a certain body, "dimension" refers to one's perspective of the universe: what we can see and what bandwidth of information we are able to perceive—in other words, a field of possibilities. People living within a specific dimension can only see what is in their range of perception.

- In the current great shift, we are changing our third density space and time limitations. This time is referred to as "the great awakening," because we are in a quantum jump of awareness and a shift in what we can perceive in our reality. The multidimensional template or field we "play in" is changing. We will transcend the limitations of our third dimension as we awaken to see more and know more.

- We are awakening from a seven-chakra system to a larger, more holistic twelve-chakra system. Until now, we had access to the seven chakras, which are our physical connection to Source energy. As we connect to larger fields of light and information, our chakra system will expand.

- The Age of Information or Age of Aquarius will bring us from third-density to fifth-density existence. We will develop and refine our higher intuitive (sixth sense) abilities such as telekinesis and psychokinesis, remote viewing skills, and instant travel.

Chapter Twelve

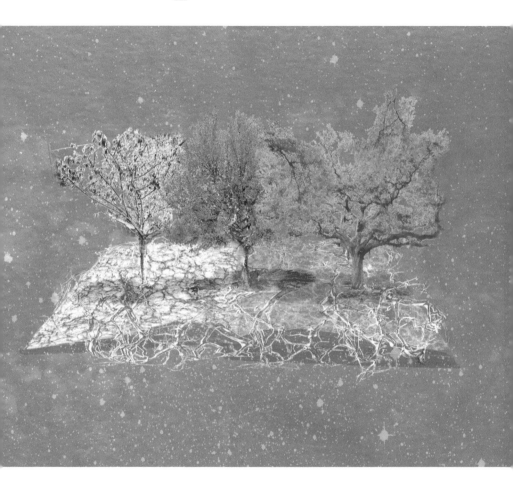

How is your consciousness impacting our future systems of global wellness?

*"Man cannot discover new oceans unless he has
the courage to lose sight of the shore."*

- Andre Gide

CHAPTER TWELVE

Creating New Systems

N ew systems must be envisioned and created when the old ones prove faulty and outdated. Our current leap in consciousness is the reason why we are seeing old structures collapse around us. Our new way of thinking no longer fits the old paradigms and systems. We are stepping out of our outdated matrix, and all the structures that went along with it.

There needs to be a restoration of Planet Earth. This will require new ways of thinking in every sector of our human existence. Educational, agricultural, urban planning, political, governmental, financial, and medical systems will all be rebuilt and upgraded, as will all aspects of how we express ourselves culturally, musically, and artistically. As we grow in consciousness, each of us will become better able to understand why we are here and connect with our unique mission.

Albert Einstein once said, "The important thing is not to stop questioning. Curiosity has its own reason for existence."[1] Humanity's need to continually ask questions will eventually bring us to a better world.

Scientific processes include questions about how things are related to each other. Most questions center on cause and effect. Astronomers work backward in time to the origins of the universe, using natural laws to explain how one force influenced another and led to the formation of galaxies, planets, and biospheres. Social scientists examine cause-and-effect connections within global systems, nations, societies, family units, and individuals. Medical science looks at bodies, systems, and organs, down to the cellular level, to discover how function and dysfunction can be explained. Energetic science deals with the flow and transformation of energy. With all these areas of potential scientific specialization, who is looking at the big picture and putting it all together?

As we realize that everything is connected, we understand that these connections determine more than just our health and well-being. It's a two-way street, or better, we abound in a multidimensional and multidirectional causal relationship with everything that exists. Outside forces are working on us, and whatever we do, whatever actions we take, also impacts the rest of the universe. An analogy that helps to explain this powerful force that connects us all is known as the Butterfly Effect. Associated with the work of the American mathematician and meteorologist Edward Lorenz, this phenomenon can be summed up by the presumption of interconnectedness such that one flap of a butterfly wing in the Amazon can cause a tornado in Texas.[2]

As we understand how more things are connected on all levels of existence, we will understand how we are affecting everything. As Johann Gottlieb Fichte wrote in *The Vocation of Man*, "You could not remove a single grain of sand from its place without thereby ... changing something throughout all parts of the immeasurable whole."

As we come to terms with how unhealthy our systems are, will we make different choices? If we take a step back without judgment and become the observer of what we have created, will we see the challenges that humanity is facing to stay healthy and well? Will we change the food we eat, the air we breathe, the water we drink, and the frequencies of our emotions? Can we begin this journey with love and acceptance?

Scientific advancement is not new. The knowledge we have about the universe we live in is constantly growing with scientific advancements, as is our understanding of the connectedness of all things. If the trend in health and wellness is going from reductionism to holism, then new studies of all the new sciences and all of their connections will follow. One study in PubMed entitled "Biofield Science: Current Physics Perspectives" states, "If biology truly derives from physics, then biology should be an extension of quantum physics, the most accurate and fundamental physical theory at our disposal."[3]

There are a number of new technologies presenting themselves already on all levels (physical, mental, and etheric), and many more will be revealed in the coming years as we enter this new Age of Aquarius. Some estimate that as many as 4,000 new inventions and technologies will come in the next ten to twenty years. Imagine how disruptive this will be to the world we know today! Already, so much new information is being revealed that it is hard for most people to keep up; in fact, many of the newest scientific breakthroughs have escaped public attention altogether.

In this chapter, we will explore some of the most meaningful new science and technologies that are based on our new understanding of frequency. These may have a vast potential impact on our ability to heal our body and function optimally within our Creator Matrix.

Transforming Science and Medicine

In this lifetime, my mission is to help support the transformation of our current medical care system into a fully integrated and holistic care system by training holistic health coaches that can contribute and nurture the process.

Our focus thus far in healthcare has been on curing disease rather than prevention and wellness, and on profit rather than people. We need to ask ourselves: is our healthcare truly serving all our needs? Yes, understanding how our cells function, how disease develops, and how the body operates every day is important; in this awareness, we can be in awe of how miraculous our bodies actually are. With this realization, we become more loving toward our bodies. However, our current disease-oriented and money-driven system has led to a one-size-fits-all approach, the very opposite of what is needed for humans to heal at all levels of body, mind, and spirit.

Many of us have begun to question the integrity of our present system and whether it truly serves humanity. The system is now changing quickly because of forced disruptions to the industry, including questioning by increasingly dissatisfied consumers. But the big-picture solution has not yet revealed itself. As a result, those of us who are committed to getting well have been forced to look for "alternative" forms of care, which can cost a great deal of personal time and financial resources. At what point will we simply say, "Enough is enough"?

In order to maintain our health in this ever-changing world, we need to update ourselves to a new reality. As human consciousness evolves, we can learn to accept and then change the things that challenge human health and wellness on both a personal and collective level. For example, I take many different supplements every day simply to feel well and healthy, and have been doing so for about twenty years. I often ask myself, "What kind of world is this? Why is it this way? Shouldn't we be getting the necessary nutrients from our food? How can it be created differently? What will we create as we learn from the new sciences?"

In this transformational time, there will be many advances in medical knowledge and techniques that will positively impact the ability of the medical world to come to the aid of patients. Our consciousness is showing us how unique we are; this will help us address health challenges through bio-individual solutions, and shift from a homogenized system to a more personalized approach. One example is how we determine what foods are best for a particular person. Until now, we have had many different theories from many different doctors, dietitians, and nutritionists as to the "perfect" diet. However, as we learn more about DNA, we can see that there is a bio-individual component that determines the best foods for a person at a particular time. This component can change as we age, as well as through life experience. We are also realizing the power of intuitive eating; as we own our Creatorship, we are learning to choose the foods that honor and nourish us. I have seen this more and more with the clients I support.

In addition to our own inner guidance systems, we may learn to rely on artificial intelligence to support bio-individual healing. New devices and apps can now determine which foods and nutrients a person needs at a particular time. In the future, AI assessment machines will become the standard of care to map out each person's unique state of being at any given moment. This will enable the discovery and development of individually targeted health solutions, as well as targeted preventative care measures. These machines are already available, but they are disruptive to the medical industry and so have not gained widespread use to date.

The ways in which we use medicine are also changing. Most people today are used to going to the doctor, receiving a diagnosis, and getting a prescription for medication to "rebalance" the body. Although medicines have served us in many ways, they are not the only answer. As we've explored in this book, the mind itself is a powerful healing tool. It has already been demonstrated that the placebo effect offers observable positive health outcomes based simply on anticipation that the person will get better. Many study participants have been given placebo pills (saline solution) in lieu of pharmaceutical treatments and yet they recovered completely against all medical odds. Some have miraculous cancer remissions and others recover from debilitating spinal injuries and walk again. The common theme is always the positive mental vision of recovery. As a nurse, I witnessed this daily. The doctor would give a diagnosis to a patient and offer a statistical percentage of survival based on "one-size-fits-all" data. The patient was often left emotionally shocked, fearful, and stressed. These low-frequency emotions and fight-or-flight responses were unhelpful for the healing process of the patient.

As you now understand after reading this book, people are more than just their biological functions and processes. We have emotions, beliefs, and inner dialogues that impact our entire system. The impact can be positive, negative, or even neutral, depending on the circumstances. Taking these additional factors into consideration goes beyond the scope of medical science today. Accepting that humans are more than just their physical bodies is the new frontier of medicine, and is where we need to go to truly help people heal and become whole.

BEYOND PHARMACOLOGY

Although medicines have their place and continue to save many lives today, the use of drugs for many chronic ailments is being challenged with our changing consciousness. Many drugs address the symptoms but not the causes of disease, and so are not truly contributing to the healing of the whole person.

Having researched the history of the medical and pharmaceutical system in the United States, I am better able to understand how we reached our current "illness-driven" system where so many solutions are pharmaceutically based. The education that supports our medical system is certainly part of the problem. In 1847, when the American Medical Association was established, there was a movement to standardize medical education. The main reason for this movement was a desire to make medical education more scientific by raising its standards and requirements. In 1893, Johns Hopkins Medical School opened its doors, and the institutionalization of scientific medicine began. The Rockefeller Institute of Medical Research was subsequently created in 1901. As research at these schools became more and more specific, and as more discoveries were made about health at the levels of systems, organs, and cells, the whole-body approaches of the past began to vanish.

In 1910, a report on medical education known as the Flexner Report was published by Abraham Flexner. The positive consequence of this report was that it helped to regulate medical school education. The backlash was that it fractured medicine into systems and took medical education further away from the holistic approach. Many schools that taught natural forms of medicine (such as osteopathy, chiropractic, and naturopathy) were not accepted as part of the new, more regulated system.

As Claire Johnson and Bart Green wrote in their 2010 article,

"100 Years After the Flexner Report: Reflections on Its Influence on Chiropractic Education" in the *Journal of Chiropractic Education*, "With the new paradigm of scientific medicine, the body began to be conceptualized in terms of systems unrelated to other systems of the body. And although specialization had been present in the context of whole-body medicine, specialization under scientific medicine began to emphasize individual systems or organs to the exclusion of the totality of the body."[4]

It has been over a hundred years since this huge change in medicine was made. The ancient wisdoms that were once commonplace but have been termed (in the previous century) "alternative" or "complementary" offer a more holistic vision of human health. Perhaps it is time to integrate some of these ancient practices with the best aspects of the modern system that we already have. One area where this could be of enormous benefit is pharmaceuticals.

For thousands of years, different cultures made use of natural plants, roots, barks, herbs, and leafy greens to make bitters and healing remedies. People learned to thrive on the diversity of what nature provided. Pharmacology has its roots in natural medicine and the use of specific plants to treat medical complaints. Many healing traditions included processes whereby the ailing person was examined in a holistic way, and remedies were devised from a perspective of body, mind, and spirit. Only in the 1880s did pharmaceutical firms in Germany begin to introduce synthetic chemicals; this has driven global research models to this day.

During my nursing training, one of the largest aspects of my education was learning about pharmaceuticals. Working as a nurse at Georgetown University, I was often (along with the other nurses) invited to join the continuing education lectures provided to medical doctors (Grand Rounds). At that time, these lectures were primarily offered by the pharmaceutical industry and usually focused on the new drugs coming on the market.

Each person is unique and reacts differently to various medications. One thing is clear: although pharmaceuticals may offer great benefits, many drugs have side effects. All drugs are subjected to animal testing in order to measure their LD50 (lethal dose 50) level, which refers to the dose at which 50 percent of individuals tested will die. Medicines are given to relieve symptoms of a disease and to change or improve the functioning of the body and mind. However, these drugs "push" the body toward a result rather than working with its natural systems and can therefore be both dangerous and toxic. In fact, prescription drugs are one of the leading causes of death (after heart disease and cancer) in the United States and Europe.[5]

I personally tend to be rather sensitive and am therefore prone to unpleasant reactions after ingesting certain medications. I have since learned to be mindful of taking a much lower dosage than prescribed. I have also learned that natural medicine (not synthetic) works better for me. I once asked a functional medicine doctor why this was, and he explained that natural medicine has a similar frequency to our bodies, whereas synthetic substances are foreign and have a completely different frequency. This made sense to me. The same consequence exists with many of the vitamin and mineral supplements on the market today; many are synthetic, made from petroleum and rocks (minerals), and are therefore toxic to humans. As pointed out by Larry Law in his book *There's an Elephant in the Room: Exposing Hidden Truths in the Science of Health*, many vitamins and minerals that are marketed as healthy for us can actually have very unhealthy effects. Take his example of calcium: "The marketing hype and deception around calcium is incredible. It actually doesn't do anything to prevent bone fractures but increases kidney stones and hardening of the arteries (atherosclerosis)."[6]

Watching the pharmaceutical industry successively promote new and emerging drugs through the years, I saw that it was hard for doctors to keep up. Being specialists to start with, and perpetually busy, they were often at a loss to choose which continuing education pathway to take to keep abreast of developments. They often lost sight of what holistic human health encompasses, while doing their very best to stay on top of it. Doctors also often need to follow certain established protocols, even if new science is questioning these protocols. This can lead to prescribing practices that are not bio-individually suited to each patient, but rather comply with established guidelines.

I do not mean to suggest that I have all the answers. No one does. We all continue to learn every day. However, as consumers look for alternatives to the chronic pharmaceutical drug use that not only alleviate symptoms but provide real solutions, we will find an integrated balance between pharmaceutical solutions and natural ones.

With the emerging uses of artificial intelligence in medicine, there is hope for a change in philosophy, especially since AI will show causes more specifically in keeping with bio-individuality. Not too far in the future, we will see that there are better ways to achieve lasting health, including more targeted medications and therapies for specific individual cases. An increasing number of doctors are becoming more open to a holistic vision of illness, health, and wellness. They are exploring more integrative approaches as well as encouraging their patients to take responsibility for their self-care. Perhaps doctors will be rewarded in the future for keeping their patients well, as opposed to simply treating symptoms and managing disease. They may even transition from being highly specialized in one area (as is the case presently) to working with each other in a multidisciplinary approach, as they cooperate and share their knowledge with each other. This is my hope, and my vision.

Environmental Challenges

Numerous documentaries and dramatic films have shown the human consequences of industrial waste. Even countries with relatively effective environmental protection legislation and monitoring mechanisms have serious pollution problems they know about—and more they don't yet know about. Pollution is a silent killer that fills the body and its vital organs with toxins to the point that cancers and other diseases result. For instance, a recent study in the *Journal of Exposure Science and Environmental Epidemiology* showed the toxicity of drinking water in the United States. Scientists from the University of New Mexico identified at least six toxic materials posing serious health risks. They noted that although the US has managed to decrease the number of bacteria in the water, chemical contaminants—including arsenic, disinfectants and their byproducts, fracking-related substances, lead, nitrate, per-and polyfluorinated alkyl substances (PFAS), and uranium, among others—have substantially increased.[7] These toxic substances have all been linked to cancer, as well as neurological and reproductive issues.

The same issues are being seen all over the world. Even the sky is not the same as it used to be. Chemtrails blanket our skies daily, but most people are not conscious of their effects. In many cities around the globe, air quality has become severely depleted.

Faced with such threats, we must first become aware as a society that our industrial structures are not supporting our optimal well-being. Then, we must take action to clean up our water supply, our food supply, and the global environment in general. Although it is probably important for everyone to detoxify their bodies on a regular basis (and I myself do a major cleanse at least once per year), individual health cannot be our only focus. We need to change the policies of our governments and health agencies. This is daunting, but it is absolutely possible.

A few years ago, I took a trip with my family to China, where it is quite common for local authorities to monitor air pollution levels and inform citizens of risk levels on any given day. In the major cities, the smog levels were very high—and, indeed, it was hard for me to take in the beauty of the Summer Palace in Beijing while also struggling to breathe. It is a great shame to realize that something as beneficial as exercise and being in nature can also become a problem when the quality of our air is compromised. A recent study published in *Elsevier*, entitled "China's improving total environmental quality and environment-economy coordination since 2000: Progress toward sustainable development goals," noted that, over the last twenty years, China's overall environmental quality has improved dramatically.[8] This finding was corroborated to me by a friend, who noticed a marked difference in air quality and smog levels since a previous trip prior to the global pandemic of 2020. Although there is a long way to go, we must all do our part to continue to make the necessary changes.

The use of synthetic chemicals in all applications is also a big concern for our health. Many plastics are noted as "endocrine disruptors," impacting optimal hormone levels in both children and adults and thereby contributing to infertility, obesity, cancer, and neurological disorders. These and other synthetic chemicals have leaked into our food and water supplies, which makes them difficult to avoid.

What are the consequences of environmental toxins for humanity in the long term? No one really knows, except that those consequences will not be positive. Each person is unique and may react differently to various toxins. Unfortunately, many of us may not feel the effects until the damage has already been done.

This information is not meant to present a doom and gloom scenario for your personal well-being. On the contrary, once you know what the dangers are, you can avoid or mitigate them. Once you know what you've been exposed to, you can take measures to ensure you are tested and/or treated to prevent major disorders. Many of these solutions are neither complex nor costly. For example, the *Journal of Agriculture and Food Chemistry*, in a 2017 study, concluded that soaking an apple for twelve to fifteen minutes in a solution of baking soda is effective in removing pesticides both on the surface and beneath the skin.[9] Awareness of what choices are good for us and the planet (organic versus conventional, natural versus synthetic, etc.) is something we can develop immediately, without too much additional effort.

Furthermore, I am convinced that new technologies and our increasing consciousness will help us solve many of these environmental issues. For example, the Ocean Cleanup Project created a flotation device in 2013, which is still helping to clean up the Great Pacific Garbage Patch without harming any part of the marine ecosystem.[10] While there is still a long way to go, these efforts bring both hope and solutions to the table. It is also possible that, as we transition to a more light-based reality, these environmental issues will heal as we heal.

The New Technologies

The new world will bring much in the form of advanced technology to support the changes I've introduced above. Scientific and technological advancement have shaken the very foundations of the old-world establishments. At this time, if we can think it, we can create it. From personalized drugs treatments to beds that can heal through frequency, health advancements are expected to release trauma, grow new tissue, and create new life stories based on bio-individuality and creativity. Changes are taking place the world over in response to innovations in food production, healthcare financing, education, and even governance.

Medical equipment is also undergoing a massive improvement, not least in response to new pandemics and the innovations arising from the challenges of military preparedness. For example, the newest medical beds are far advanced beyond traditional models. Tele-medicine solutions provide access to those in remote locations without access to expert clinicians. New rule-based ventilators were introduced in the aftermath of Covid-19 that can be operated by non-expert medical support staff. As previously mentioned, AI-enabling infrastructure and data collection technologies are already improving diagnostics and specialized care. Computer advances, digitalization, and automation have improved just about every aspect of medical care, including upgrades for hospital rooms, beds, and other equipment; modernized ambulances and emergency rooms; more refined blood banks and laboratories; and evolved antiseptics and anesthesia. This list is long.

As discussed in earlier chapters, the field of energy medicine—which deals with therapeutic applications of our energy field—is also evolving quickly. Our energetic field is now recognized as being a powerful force that influences our vitality, state of being, and well-being. These energy fields specifically impact the life force of our biological systems, organs, and cells.

On my YouTube channel, I interview many people involved in energy medicine healing. These doctors and therapists help people heal by not only addressing their physical and mental well-being, but also by attending to their energetic imbalances. Respected fields of study like homeopathy, cranial-osteopathy, reflexology, reconnective healing, kinesiology, yoga, meditation, and acupuncture/acupressure address health by bringing into balance the different energy fields.

There are also a growing number of psychological/emotional modalities that help the client reprogram the subconscious and rebalance emotions and trauma. Several of the most well-known are Psych-K, EFT (Emotional Freedom Techniques), NLP (Neuro Linguistic Programming), the Silva Ultramind System, Biofield Tuning (sound therapy), The Journey, and Pesso Boyden System Psychomotor (PBSP). All of these methods help to shift outdated belief systems and low-frequency emotions that are blocking energy channels, release traumas of all kinds, and create a more positive, cohesive working nervous system and balanced energetic system within all areas of the Creator Matrix. In an article entitled "Six pillars of energy medicine: clinical strengths of a complementary paradigm," David Feinstein, PhD writes: "Conventional medicine, at its foundation, focuses on the biochemistry of cells, tissue, and organs. Energy medicine, at its foundation, focuses on the fields that organize and control the growth and repair of cells, tissues, and organs and on ways of influencing those fields." In this article he describes how the six pillars show "why the energy paradigm is rapidly gaining strength among healthcare practitioners."[11] He offers clinical examples such as working with MS patients by massaging energy points that can "[bring] about changes in the disease process rather than ... symptom suppression of most MS treatments."

I myself have found modalities like The Journey helpful at clearing emotional blockages because they address the emotional, physical, mental, and spiritual root causes. The Journey was founded by Brandon Bays and her husband, Kevin Billet. Bays began sharing her techniques after mastering her own healing journey with them.[12] My family and I have found this technique, in combination with kinesiology, to be very helpful in healing the Creator Matrix and reprogramming the subconscious.

Research on these new modalities is in its early stages, but the number of enthusiasts is increasing as positive anecdotal evidence points to vast potential. Also, research into these innovations requires significant investments of time and resources, without guarantees for return on investment; with monetary incentives being low, progress has been slow. However, slow doesn't equal nonexistent, and promising new insights abound. For example, if someone in a difficult marriage develops an autoimmune disease, practitioners may no longer choose only prescription medications, but may also recommend seeing a functional medicine doctor, taking sessions with a therapist or coach, or improving the patient's mental outlook through practices such as jogging, dancing, meditation, qi gong, tai chi, or yoga.

As we witness our system changing from disease-based to well-ness-based, everything we do in the current medical system will be transformed. There will be a great transition to frequency-based energy medicine as we continue to learn and integrate the new sciences with a holistic understanding of body, mind, and spirit, and adapt to a more multidimensional way of living. As Nikola Tesla predicted, "The day science begins to study non-physical phenomena, it will make more progress in one decade than in all the previous centuries of its existence. To understand the true nature of the universe, one must think in terms of energy, frequency, and vibration."[13]

As we increase our personal frequency through this ascension process, new technologies working with the expanded quantum field will support us to adjust to higher frequency levels by rebalancing and bringing harmony to the body, mind, and spirit matrix. I have inter-viewed several people who have invented technologies that work with the quantum field healing frequencies. The Harmonic Egg, the Blu Room, the Energy Enhancement System, and Medical Bed devices are available now, to name but a few. In the coming years, I expect this quantum field of energetic medicine to explode with hundreds of new technologies.

I had the pleasure of interviewing Gail Lynn, inventor of the Harmonic Egg and author of *Unlocking the Ancient Secrets of Healing*.

After experiencing severe health challenges, Gail sought out more holistic solutions to her problem. The Harmonic Egg uses a "sacred geometry chamber" that, through sound and light with unique bio-individual frequencies, releases blocked energy by rerouting the system to be more in flow. Testimonials from those who have used the Harmonic Egg show that it has helped to relieve stress and pain, speed up the rate of recovery, improve clarity and focus, create spiritual and emotional restoration, and support better general health.[14] I have personally used this system and experienced many healing moments. For instance, I suffered with neck pain for decades, but after making positive intentions within the Harmonic Egg I was finally able to heal. I have not experienced neck pain since. I also noticed that making any kind of intention in the Egg accelerated my ability to manifest in general.

Another new technology grounded in frequency-based medicine is the Blu Room, invented by J.Z. Knight and co-developed by Dr. Matthew Martinez. It uses narrowband UV-B light, sound therapy, and sacred geometry, as well as the individual's intention, to increase a person's frequency and therefore improve their well-being.[15] Users of the Blu Room have experienced a range of benefits from deep relaxation, improved cellular healing, and increased spiritual connection and development. Others have observed relief from physical pain, mental stress, and anxiety, as well as faster healing and greater consciousness.

The Energy Enhancement System, invented and developed by Dr. Sandra Rose Michael, PhD, DNM, DCSJL, uses custom-installed computers to generate morphogenic energy fields—aka, scalar waves—which "return the body to a more original and appropriate electrical matrix" and promote cellular rejuvenation. This system has been recognized by dozens of medical and scientific professional conferences around the world.[16]

MedBed (medical bed) technologies also use quantum healing through radiation, vibrations, sound waves, and thought waves. This technology offers detoxification, anti-aging, cellular regeneration, and healing.[17]

I have recently come across a type of healing that I find extremely promising. It is called the Zone Technique. Dr. Peter Goldman, who has refined the technique, was greatly influenced by Dr. Thurman Fleet, who created Zone Therapy in 1931. As a chiropractor, Dr. Goldman learned that misaligned spinal vertebrae can negatively affect nerve flow, which is the root cause of disease; therefore, realignment of the vertebrae can restore health. The Zone Technique takes this foundation of healing further by restoring signals between the brain, spinal cord, and body systems for amazing healing results.[18] All of these technologies reconnect and rebalance our human energy fields to the quantum field of pure light and coherence.

I always encourage my students and clients to experience any of these new energy healing modalities that call to them. It can also be helpful to go to therapists who practice Reconnective Healing, the Zone Technique, and the Journey, to name a few. Meeting with therapists or trained coaches who can help reprogram the subconscious may also be a wonderful way to get started on a healing journey. What is important is to have the courage to try something new. With courage, we can experience the benefits to our health by caring for our Creator Matrix in new ways.

SELF-HEALING

Many years ago, I received a call from a friend, Henriette. She had discovered a lump in her breast. Within days, she was diagnosed with an aggressive form of triple-negative cancer. Henriette is an energy healer and knows a lot about the mental, emotional, and spiritual influences that impact holistic healing. However, she later shared with me that, during her two years of recovery from that cancer, she needed to learn to connect with and listen to the needs of her body in a much deeper way. In the past, she had always been more focused on the spiritual and emotional aspects of healing; now, she learned to truly ground her spirit in her body.

As there was urgency to do the surgery after her diagnosis, Henriette did it as soon as possible. The lump was removed, and in the subsequent weeks she was able to connect with what she calls her "golden space of deep knowingness." She also found a clinic in Switzerland that offered her an alternative to chemotherapy and radiation. Over the next two years, she was given holistic treatments that combined deeply cleansing the body (removing heavy metals) with high amounts of nutrition (vitamins, minerals, and glycans) and antioxidants (vitamin C infusions). Henriette also received holistic dental treatment to remove toxic mercury fillings and open the channels of blocked meridians. However, one of the most profound treatments for her was hyperthermia. The clinical machine put her body in a high-fever state to help boost her white blood cell count and immune response.

I'm grateful to say that Henriette has been in remission for nearly ten years and is happier and healthier than ever.

During this acceleration of consciousness, many people are often choosing the natural route of self-healing for common diseases. What is important is that each person follows their inner knowingness to choose methods of healing that resonate with them. Each person must decide for themselves what they will allow in their healing journey. As discussed, our beliefs matter; what we give our power to will influence the outcome. What is important is to respect every person's choice as being the right one for them.

With all the new technologies and inventions available (and still to come), our options for healing modalities will expand and change. Simply connecting to the quantum field brings a larger bandwidth of frequency that can accelerate self-healing, and in many cases produce spontaneous and immediate healing. As mentioned before, I learned Reconnective Healing many years ago, and I am amazed at how quickly it helps raise my frequencies and rebalance my system when I'm feeling unwell. I am convinced that, with the help of these new modalities and technologies, we will all be able to access the field and heal ourselves instantly in the future.

Our transformation to a more "well-based" health system will also change the way we think about disease. "Disease" has been ingrained in our subconscious as an inevitable part of life. Many people believe that, if we live long enough, we will eventually get a disease of some kind. This thought that we live our lives and then get sick is something we must change. Disease is not an inevitability, but a programmed belief that we, as individuals and as a collective, manifest repeatedly. This thought pattern must be reprogrammed in order for us to live our lives to the fullest and be well and balanced at the same time. Remember, thoughts are energetic waves of information that mold plasma in the Universal Field to manifest in the physical. So, why not hold the thought, "I get stronger and healthier with each year I live?"

As previously discussed, everything is energy and has an energetic field. Understanding this will make it possible for us to heal not just our physical bodies, but everything in our reality. What if we could "heal" and repair our businesses, physical possessions, systems, and governments just by tapping into the proper frequencies? Some have called this information Intrinsic (Informational) Data Fields (IDFs). The quantum field is omnipotent or all-knowing because it contains "all that is." Therefore, everything needed to heal is already there.

Let us take a deeper look at the energetic phenomena of IDFs and how they will transform our view of health and wellness. According to wellness coach Norianna Diesel, our perception is only possible because we observe and interpret energy waves of different frequencies in our surroundings. Our human bodies radiate and absorb this energy. This creates the illusion that our physical world is solid. Yet, science is showing us that the base of everything is mostly empty space and energetic light fields. Ms. Diesel clarifies the relationship between Intrinsic Data Fields and energy in this way: "It is this energy that is constantly being shaped by IDFs. As we progress in our scientific understanding of reality, we are realizing more and more that our health and well-being are ultimately tied into the 'healthy' function of the data exchange between Informational Data Fields and the energy that fuels our bodies."[19]

To summarize, if these IDFs are misinterpreted or the perception of these fields is misread, the problem lies in the exchange between IDFs and our own energy. We cannot read information clearly if we are not well-connected to the field. Compare this to our computers not being connected to electricity or the Internet, and therefore being unable to access the information necessary for our work.

As we've explored throughout this book, the ability of our physical bodies to connect to multidimensional fields of existence seems to depend on cellular well-being at the physical level. The field of glycoscience will lead the way in understanding cells' ability to communicate. As we discussed in Chapter Nine, no communication between cells takes place without glycans, and therefore nothing can happen in the body without glycans. In the future, as we study the science of glycans, we will better understand the connection between glycans and the Universal Field, and the nature of the communication between the two. This will help us to understand all aspects of multidimensional communication.

As mentioned before, many research organizations and tech companies, like Glycan Age, are trying to understand the different combinations of these glycans and their influence on communication in the body. Glycan Age can evaluate the glycan codes in a person's cells to see personal differences in their individual health as well as potential vulnerabilities toward certain diseases. Soon, healing by working with glycans will be the new normal, and self-healing through managing glycans will likewise be widespread.

Change is the New Game

The world is not what we once believed it to be. Therefore, we are being asked to let go of old belief systems. This process requires change. As we let go of the old, we are asking ourselves what is real, what is truth, why am I here, where am I going, and what is life on Planet Earth really all about? These questions often present themselves as a crisis of identity and purpose.

Many of our old belief systems are tied up with past traumas and low-frequency emotions. These old belief systems have created patterns over lifetimes and generations. Many of our belief systems have been driving us karmically. As mentioned in Chapter Eleven, karma is distorted thought patterns that have become stuck at the cellular and subconscious levels throughout the Creator Matrix. These thought patterns are like dark cobwebs sticking to the memory matrix of our cells, driving and influencing our manifestations. When we want to make change, we have to change—and what we have to change are our thoughts.

It is impossible to change a habit or behavioral pattern without releasing and letting go of the thoughts at its base. Most of these old networks of thoughts are directly connected to low-frequency emotions, fears, and specific storylines. As we learned in the first part of this book, when a thought is connected to an emotion and/or storyline in the subconscious, it is very powerful. It can completely run a person's life if they are unaware. If the distorted thought pattern complex is not recognized, it is impossible to create lasting change. Many people try to attract new things into their life without changing the thoughts that caused the old things to appear. If the wound is extreme enough, it is called a trauma. When people have a trauma, they need professional help from a psychiatrist, psychologist, or a trained trauma therapist. However, if a person wants to change a habit or an old belief system, they can work effectively with a coach.

THE ROLE OF HEALTH AND WELLNESS COACHING

Most of us want to feel good, find a fulfilling life path, and enjoy a healthy mental and physical state. However, many are also struggling with stress-related diseases, debilitating addictions, poor quality of health, and/or the greatest health crises of our time, obesity. The need for change is there; however, until now, our systems have not supported change. This situation fueled the rise of health and wellness coaching as early as the 1990s. Today, the title of "Certified Health Coach" has become one of the most sought-after in the world. Many professionals in medicine and other fields are seeking out this education to add coaching skills to their repertoire and learn more holistic applications for this existing knowledge and qualifications. Health and wellness coaches, through motivational interviewing and behavior change theories, coach their clients to make changes in all areas of life that improve and affect their well-being. This holistic skill set that offers one-on-one care seems to be one of the missing pieces of our current healthcare system. Rising levels of stress, poor food quality, toxic environment, sedentary lifestyle, and poor lifestyle choices are propelling the need for change in the medical system, and health and wellness coaches are proving to be a vital part of the change.

Health and wellness coaches help people reflect on areas of their lives that they want to change. All areas that affect well-being can be the focus of a coaching session. Health and wellness coaching helps clients realize the power of their role as a Creator in the present moment. The health coach rarely looks at the client's past for change, but rather focuses the coaching conversation on the here and now. Coaching conversations are always client-driven and are often one-on-one sessions whereby the coach and client co-create (weekly) goals and action steps for change. The health and wellness coach acts as a mirror to help guide the client toward self-reflection and self-recognition, and to help them connect to areas of their lives that may need attention and reconnection. By working with people uniquely and individually, coaches can offer a new perspective as to how clients are living their lives and highlight opportunities for change. Then, they can support clients with lifestyle habits by helping them with (secondary) food choices and other related habits. This is much like a "rebooting" of the system, helping the body, mind, and spirit matrix to function optimally at all levels.

Our choices influence the direction of our life and happiness. Choices in life reinforce our control over the circumstances of our lives and the lives of those around us. The coaching process is centered on the client's agenda and, when successful, empowers the client with tools and perspectives that enable them to consciously regain control of their health and wellness. Prior to the coaching moment, they may have felt out of control or like they were victims of their own life story.

Their lifestyle choices and habits were influenced by the perspective and emotions they had at the time. As the client learns to move away from a "victim consciousness," they can feel more in control and step into their authentic power as the Creators they truly are. When this happens, their emotions may feel more expanded and they may operate from a higher frequency, which will positively influence their state of being, life direction, and certainly their life story. On a physical level, living from this higher frequency will optimally affect their cellular well-being and energetic flow.

Coaching can also be an effective way of learning to come to grips with emotions. Many people get stuck in their story and the emotions associated with it. This can influence their state of being and critical life choices in ways they never realize. Their state of being (frequency) can even limit the possibilities of what choices they can imagine. When we are feeling down, we often cannot "see" any positive solutions; well-trained coaches, through listening skills and reflective questioning, can help a client change the direction and frequency that they are "hanging out" in. I have helped many people to forgive themselves and forgive others to clear stagnant energy and change direction. Professional psychotherapy is also an option for those whose emotional state is blocked from trauma, and many therapists can also offer personalized recommendations for improved health and well-being.

A Wellness Revolution

Humanity has witnessed many revolutions for freedom and basic rights. These revolutions were and are about slavery, about racism and discrimination, about the right to vote for women and minorities, and about the right to decent and safe working conditions. Although we must continue to improve these areas, what the world needs now, in our time, is a wellness revolution. As each of us wakes up in the morning, we need to feel well so that we are able to participate in life with our full attention and high consciousness. We need to start to "feel great" on all levels, transitioning away from trauma and illness.

Learning to heal ourselves within the Creator Matrix will simultaneously empower us to heal our systems, institutions, and governments so that they can function in keeping with a fifth-density reality of love and transparency. It will be an all-encompassing ripple effect, as everything is connected.

We need a people's movement that emerges from the bottom up and helps people to make the necessary changes to transform unhealthy habits into positive and self-serving habits. Many things will be discovered during this new time of awakening about human health and wellness. It is an amazing time to be alive!

Chapter Summary

- Due to our current leap in consciousness, old structures are collapsing around us, old paradigms and systems no longer fit, and our present matrix is outdated. We are asked to create new structures in every sector of our human existence, based on new ways of thinking.

- Everything is connected in a multidimensional and multidirectional causal relationship with everything that exists. Whatever action we take impacts the whole. By making these changes we will create a ripple effect throughout our world and universe.

- Our current healthcare system is transforming from a disease-oriented, one-size-fits-all approach to a wellness-oriented, bio-individual system. With these changes we are moving from a reductionist approach to a holistic one.

- We are moving toward a more holistic healthcare setting where our current medical system will be integrated with ancient forms of natural medicine. Natural medicine has a similar frequency to our bodies.

- As we increase our personal frequency through this ascension process, new technologies working with the expanded quantum field will support us as we adjust to higher frequency levels by rebalancing and bringing harmony back to the body, mind, and spirit matrix.

- We are transitioning to frequency-based energy medicine with new technologies that work with the quantum field of healing frequencies, like the Harmonic Egg, the Blu Room, the Energy Enhancement System, and Medical Bed devices, and many more to come. Connecting to the quantum field brings a larger bandwidth of frequency that can accelerate self-healing, and in many cases produce spontaneous and immediate healing.

- New technologies and our increasing consciousness will help us resolve and clean up many environmental challenges, like toxins in our water and food supply, air pollution, the use of pesticides, and endocrine-disrupting synthetic chemicals like plastics.

- In order to create change and attract new things into our lives, we need to start transforming our thoughts that attracted the old. Health and wellness coaches help people to reflect on areas of their lives that they want to change, and to make change happen.

- We need a wellness revolution, a people's movement that emerges from the bottom up and helps humanity transform.

- This is an amazing time to be alive!

Chapter Thirteen

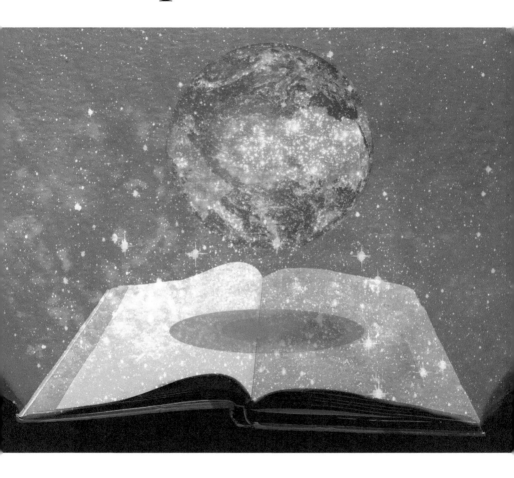

*How are we awakening
to the New Earth?*

"The real revolution is the evolution of consciousness."

- Anonymous

CHAPTER THIRTEEN

The New Earth

One day this past summer, my brother Jim and I had a special moment together. It had been several years since I was able to go back home to the United States due to the pandemic, so I greatly appreciated this time with my large family.

My brother shared with me a vision that happened to him as he was in therapy. As I listened to him describe his experience, I was struck by how powerful it was as a metaphor for our work as a co-Creator in the New Earth.

Jim was taken on a journey inside his brain. He was looking at and experiencing his own neural pathways. He was shown how limited, rigid, and habitual his thought patterns had become, and how few neural networks he was using every day. He then saw a black space with eighteen columns that were softly lit. Each column represented a thought in his brain. The experience was much like being in a pinball machine, as the ball ricocheted off of these eighteen thoughts over and over again. As the journey progressed, rows of columns began to appear behind the original eighteen. He became excited that his thoughts were expanding. After a few layers of columns had appeared, light penetrated from behind the last rows; eventually, the light blocked the columns, and all he saw was light. Within moments of that expansion, the light took over the darkness, and the columns began to fade.

At the end of this journey, light was all he saw—light, and himself, sitting cross-legged in silhouette. He felt surrounded by universal wholeness and was astonished by how expanded and powerful he had become through this process. He felt freer, lighter, and more creative. This expansion process helped him feel joy and feel more himself. It was as if he'd been stuck in a maze, and he was now finally free.

Jim's vision illustrates the challenge of adapting to our highest potential, stepping into our power to become a Creator, and co-creating our reality. If we want to claim our power as a Creator, we need to move away from the familiar, and into the unknown.

Beyond Suffering and Judgment

As human beings, we are all the same at our core. We are all searching for safety, connection, love, and fulfillment. Learning that we can choose what happens, and how we react to what happens, is fundamental to our ability to step into and own our true power as a co-Creator.

As I reflect on the changes we must make to prepare ourselves for the New Earth, I see that many of our patterns and thought forms must change. The first and most important is the thought that we can only learn through suffering. As we each have our challenges and life lessons, many might say, "When we suffer, we grow." This is reflected in the Buddhist saying, "No mud, no lotus." But could it be possible to grow without this kind of suffering? As more and more people wake up to the power of their own Creatorship, perhaps we will be able to take responsibility for our life stories, thoughts, belief systems, and choices, and realize we can do this without suffering. I have observed spiritual masters walking on hot coals and sharing that they were not burned and did not feel pain. This was because they held a strong belief that there would be no pain. For them, suffering was a choice, and they chose not to feel it.

Suffering has served a purpose, of course: it has given us an opportunity to get deeply into our stories, to develop compassion for ourselves and others, and help us make sudden changes to our life stories that no longer serve us. These life stories we suffer through show us something profound and bring us into contact with parts of ourselves that we have denied, ignored, or judged. In suffering, we feel emotions like disappointment, sadness, loss, low self-esteem, and lack intensely. By changing our story, we have an opportunity to self-reflect and choose a new path, a new direction, one where we have integrated the lessons from this past story. However, this change is dependent on our *awareness*, not on our suffering. We can choose to have one without the other.

Another pattern that would be helpful to change is our propensity to judge ourselves and others. I have come to understand that what we judge we will continue to interact with. Our judgments act like a mirror showing us what we have not yet accepted and loved within ourselves. We can carry judgments for many reasons, including learned behavior and genetic karma as well as our wounded ego. Our DNA can carry more than just medical and genetic tendencies like blue eyes and cancer. As already discussed in this book, it can carry genetically stuck emotions and belief systems as well as imbalances and traumas. When we realize this, we can heal these imbalances and see others' perspectives. When we feel whole from within, we develop compassion for ourselves, others, and their stories. We can let go of judgments and simply let things be as they are.

That said, it is not possible to change another person's story without it being their choice. We cannot tell someone to love themselves, tell them to heal, or tell them to choose another path. When we do so, we take away their Creatorship and infringe on their free will. And most of the time, when we try to do this, it's because we have not yet claimed our own role as a Creator and are trying to force an outcome through the actions and experiences of others. Only when you do the work of claiming Creatorship for yourself will you be in a position to guide others toward the same. Everyone is the Creator of their own story, whether they have chosen it consciously or unconsciously. Each soul needs the story that they chose, as it serves their soul's journey.

Realizing that we can decide not to suffer and not to judge is a powerful step toward creating the loving New Earth we are all seeking. In the new world, instead of judging, we will learn to discern.

DISCERNMENT

Where judgment is based on "right" and "wrong", discernment is our ability to choose what we do and do not allow in our personal energy field and life story. Judgments are often based on our limited beliefs and the illusion of duality. When we become more conscious and reprogram these beliefs, we will learn to be Creators, and consequently be able to discern without judgment what we want to get involved with and what we don't, what is good for us and what is not.

Although humankind has always grappled with the concept of telling myth from reality and fact from fallacy, this particular form of discernment has never been more complicated than in the present era of "fake news." As we present futuristic technologies, as I have done earlier in this book, some ideas might seem closer to science fiction than science, and more like fantasy than fact. Oftentimes the array of new and incredible ideas and concepts can be bewildering and mind-boggling. As a result, you may be tempted to judge what you have read. I ask you instead to discern. Only you can decide if this information serves your soul and your evolution as a Creator.

Where do you draw the line with your levels of trust and skepticism? This is again where we need to develop and learn to use our intuition. Many parts of the old world need to adapt to new ways of thinking. Many structures will fall in the years to come, and many will be transformed. Learning that we create our reality through thoughts will change everything. Disruption of the status quo can be effective in bringing about needed change. As Arthur Schopenhauer wrote, "Every original idea is first ridiculed, then vigorously attacked, and finally taken for self-evident."

Perhaps, in this new world that we are creating, it is best to question everything. The world is evolving so quickly at this time, and because our consciousness is expanding, we will begin to see more, know more, and understand more. As we are awakening, the world we thought we once knew and trusted will crumble, leaving many of us feeling confused, angry, uncertain, and uncomfortable. This is already happening, and it will continue throughout this ascension. We will all face shocking truths about our reality that will challenge our belief systems and our very way of life—if not now, then soon. That is why it is important for each soul to remain optimistic. With all the change that is happening, I have learned to become more open-minded and question everything that I used to believe. Creating a free and truly holistic society will take time and a great deal of collective patience. Remember that we own our story, and others own theirs. This will help us to become more accepting of what others choose to experience.

Learning to practice discernment is learning to choose what you put your energy toward as a Creator. If you can think it, you can create it. Imagine the possibilities.

CREATE YOUR OWN SAFE SPACE

Creating a feeling of safety in our shifting world can be a challenge for each of us. As we clear blockages on all levels of our Creator Matrix and begin to fully integrate our body, mind, and spirit, it will be essential for each of us to create safety in any situation we choose to inhabit. We will choose safety over fear.

By stepping into our full power as a Creator, we take full responsibility for what we choose to create. Learning to discern what is safe for us and what is not will become more obvious and much easier. As we grow in consciousness, we will develop the awareness to create safety in any situation. A two-year-old doesn't understand that it is dangerous to run into the street, but a ten-year-old does. As we grow in awareness, we will understand what stories we want to get involved with and which stories we will avoid. We will also learn to use our energetic field to transmute energy to feel safe even in uncertain circumstances.

Spiritual Awakening, Changing Relationships

As we change, so too will our relationships. Stepping into our power as divine Creators will lead us to become more authentic, independent, and sovereign. Our relationships with ourselves will change first. Many refer to this change as a "spiritual awakening."

Going through this many years ago, I felt very alone and disconnected from all that I previously felt connected to, yet excited to realize that there was more to this earthly life than I ever imagined. Although I knew that I was a spiritual being who was temporarily here in a physical body, my awakening gave me a greater sense of purpose and a remembrance of who I really am and who we all are. We are powerful, part of pure consciousness, and able to shape our reality.

I also experienced physical symptoms during this time, as if the awakening process was happening on all levels of mind, body, and spirit. I felt pain and discomfort in places that needed love, attention, and release. I had more lucid dreams, intermittent insomnia, heightened sensitivity, and acceleration of psychic awareness. My clients have also reported experiencing depression, anxiety, skin irritations, dizziness, ear buzzing (tinnitus), digestive issues, heart palpitations, increased connection to nature, more intuitive observation of beliefs/habits/self-dialogue, and excitement for life itself. Most of the time, there is a feeling of hitting rock-bottom; some refer to this as "the dark night of the soul." This darkness is the beginning of the process of rebirth, and many who experience this never fear their shadow side again. Rather, their "darkness" integrates with a much higher perspective that goes above duality.

People who have experienced a spiritual awakening and raised their frequency may discover that many of their long-term relationships no longer serve them. As we allow change, so will our environment change, and our relationships are part of that. As we grow in consciousness, we will learn to discern which of our relationships are for a reason, a season, or a lifetime. Some are true heart/soul connections, some are there for us to learn a lesson, and some are simply temporary and serve our creative storylines at a moment in time. As we awaken, we will start to recognize relationships that are deep soul connections from many lives. As we are healing, some of our relationships may need healing too. Ultimately, the most profound healing between two people comes through acceptance and forgiveness.

Here's an example: I once knew a woman who found out her husband was cheating on her. For many people this would seem like the end; however, the woman decided that she had two options. The first was to allow her anger to overtake her and ask him to leave immediately and forever. The second was to share her pain concerning the deceit and work toward forgiveness. Out of the initial confrontation, she decided to offer him the time and space to explore his feelings for this other woman and look at why he cheated in the first place. Eventually, giving him this freedom and understanding opened a door to a deeper connection between the two of them. He broke up with the other woman soon thereafter, realizing that he had been searching for more excitement and connection within his own marriage and had been unable to express this. Because of this experience and how they handled it, the two of them were able to change their story and therefore their future timeline. They were able to heal the animosity between them and move on to another level of consciousness and relationship. If she had made a different decision and chosen the first option, the story, emotions, and divisions could have changed both of their fates, and perhaps even created deep imbalances in their physical expression.

Many times, after death, divorce, or other major relationship shifts, people manifest imbalances that lead to disease. Now, of course, there is no "right" or "wrong"—sometimes, divorce or other drastic measures are necessary to our continued growth. Not all relationships will last a lifetime, but how we handle the relationships will make a difference in how we evolve and how the storylines we choose play out in our Creator Matrix. By resolving their story in a positive way, the couple above were able to avoid accumulating energetic blockages or lingering low-frequency emotions. In my life, when relationships become conflictual, I remember that I allowed the present situation and had a part in creating it. This allows me to find gratitude for the story, no matter how it ends.

FORGIVENESS AND GRATITUDE

When we experience our life stories in challenging ways and/or have unresolved karmic storylines, we can create distorted thought patterns that can sit in our DNA and block our energy fields. We need to digest our stories in order to rid ourselves of these blockages. Many times, this means finding a measure of forgiveness and gratitude for ourselves and the people involved.

When we cannot forgive, the issue remains unresolved. This keeps energetic spiritual cords active as well as all the stuck emotions between people. There are many different ideas about what forgiveness means and how we can achieve it. In Greek, *aphiem* means to pardon, to remit as an offense or debt, or to overlook an offense;[1] this is the definition I like best for forgiveness.

When we forgive, we become free of distorted thought patterns and cut energetic cords that are draining our life force. Having released someone from their debt or offense to us, or let them go, we become free. A preacher once explained to me that forgiveness is not the same as forgetting. It is harder to forget, even if we want to: since everything is stored in the Akash, once we have been hurt, the pain and all related emotions will also be stored, along with what these experiences have taught us. However, as we forgive, we release the stored emotions and transmute the darkness, keeping only the lessons learned.

We can all learn to transmute the lower frequencies of anger, resentment, and hatred to the very high frequency of gratitude. This gratitude can extend to both the story and to all those who participated in it. This comes easier as we grow in consciousness and learn to see from a higher perspective. Connecting to the frequency of gratitude for everything and everyone we encounter can shift our frequency instantly. Sometimes, to release, forgive, and find gratitude may require a spiritual ceremony. We can also choose to work with a therapist who can facilitate consciously speaking to the higher soul of the other. Eventually, we can learn to shift this perspective on our own.

The illusion, of course, is that we must wait for the other to forgive us (or repent of their actions) in order for us to be free or move on. What is important is that we thank them for the story, cut the energetic cords, and realize that everyone played their role for the benefit of duality and the evolution of consciousness. If we refuse to forgive, our energetic field and light body will become heavier. These energetic blockages can be carried from lifetime to lifetime and passed on through our genetics. Everyone who truly forgives and also forgives themselves will feel lighter, learn the lesson, and transcend the karmic story.

True forgiveness brings a feeling of tremendous peace to our souls. The New Earth will bear witness to this level of healing throughout mankind.

Heart Consciousness, Love, and Cooperation

As we become Creators of our stories, we will master them. We will learn to live from our hearts in a state of unconditional love and acceptance of all that is. With a more expanded consciousness, we will make different decisions. When we learn to function from a state of abundance and let go of any feelings of lack within each part of our Creator Matrix, all areas will begin to thrive. As we will no longer be functioning in a collective survival mode, humanity will make more ethical choices that serve both the individual and the collective from a higher perspective.

We will instantly be able to connect to the universe and the quantum field of infinite possibilities through the electromagnetic fields of our hearts. Some masters have referred to this field as "superconsciousness," a field of all-knowing and all-loving. Our hearts will become more aligned with our true self and our Creator Matrix will become "coherent". Coherence comes from the Latin word that means "to stick together." According to the definition of coherence, "When something has *coherence*, all of its parts fit together well."[2] As all aspects of our Creator Matrix become integrated together, our heart fields will expand, and we will be able to step into our authentic power as Creators.

This is such an exciting time to be alive! Each soul that is awakening will come to understand the significance of the transition that we are making to a New Earth and fifth-density living. Until now, we have been living in a world of conflict and competition; when we come from a state of unconditional love, we can create a world of cooperation. As we rise above duality, we will be able to see the beauty of living cooperatively. Each of us will step into our own sovereignty and hold higher and higher frequencies of light and love. Cooperation will be necessary for the complete restoration and healing of Mother Earth, as well as our individual bodies and minds.

A NEW UNDERSTANDING OF COMPASSION

The propensity to make certain life choices at certain moments reflects our bio-individuality, emotions, health, well-being, and numerous other variables. Self-awareness, and awareness of the differences between ourselves and others, opens the door to a certain degree of acceptance.

Let's face it, we all have certain inclinations and proclivities that determine our preferences. These preferences could be in relation to food, work, leisure, relationships, or any number of life choices. When we can completely accept ourselves and others as we are, with all our differences and imperfections, we will have uncovered the keystone of compassion.

Ushering in this new time on Earth requires a more conscious definition of compassion. We used to look at compassion as a need to interfere with the stories of others. When we had compassion, what we really had was pity and concern for others who were suffering. When we had sympathy, we had feelings for someone's misfortune. When we felt empathy, we could feel what the other was feeling, positive or negative. As a result, many of us felt an obligation to interfere as a way of "helping." As we become the conscious Creators of our stories, we do not need to take on the responsibility of someone's life or story anymore. The new definition of compassion is to allow the other their Creatorship by allowing them to direct their own story, and only offer help when we are asked to do so.

When I learned about this new definition of compassion, I had been so programmed to feel responsible to help and "fix" everyone that it was difficult for me to step back, let go, and realize that not everyone was ready for change. Some people still needed their stories, and many times it was uncomfortable to watch their process as they continued to suffer, but their story was not mine to change. Learning that each Creator chooses and needs their story has liberated me from this responsibility.

This new boundary is one reason why health and wellness coaching is so important. Everything in a session is client-driven. In other words, good coaches allow their clients their own storylines. They allow the client to make changes, new goals, and action plans at their own pace and in their own unique way.

ACCEPTANCE, JOY, AND HUMOR

During difficult times, when there seemed to be little hope, I would often ask questions of my spiritual teachers. One particular teacher would respond to my questions with more questions. She would ask, "What would happen if you just accepted the situation as it is?" At first, I could not imagine accepting as I was caught up in resistance, uncertainty, and pain. However, as I learned to accept whatever was showing up that I did not like, I learned a powerful skill. Immediately, through complete acceptance, all resistance and fear would vanish, and I would be led to feel the opposite emotion, love.

While love is the answer to all suffering, laughter is the greatest medicine! The ability to find humor in all experiences is a true gift. I am grateful to have been given this powerful example through my family and family-in-law. Some are so gifted at using humor that they are able to lighten any situation, even challenging ones. My husband is particularly good at this, which has helped me so much during very challenging moments. Many more of my family also use humor as a way to transmute and change the energy instantly, raising the frequency for both themselves and others. What a co-creation! Laughter is a powerful and contagious connecting force. Humor and laughter can offer a tremendous shift in perspective; you simply cannot be laughing and feel lower-frequency emotions like anger and sadness at the same time. I have also noticed how quickly using humor can bring us to a feeling of gratitude for the experience, and how it can expedite our path toward acceptance. I myself have used laughter consciously to provide comfort, bring joy, and help unify groups of people. I encourage you to smile, laugh, play, and find joy consciously each day as you learn to shift your energy into lighter and higher frequencies.

Our Awakening Communication Networks

The shift that we are making now will be reflected in our DNA. As we make these evolutionary steps, we are expanding and activating more strands of DNA. As we discussed earlier in this book, we have been using a limited bandwidth of two strands of DNA for eons. We already know from epigenetics that we can change our DNA and that our thoughts, words, and beliefs also impact it. Therefore, we are changing our DNA every day. In glycoscience we learned that the cells are multidimensional and connect to fields of information in order to communicate. Now science is beginning to look at the communication network of DNA. Spiritual scientist Linda Gadbois, while looking at DNA and how it communicates, stated, "DNA is actually composed of a liquid crystalline substance that acts as a form of antenna, receiver, and transmitter of holographic information. It's constantly in the process of taking in information from its environment and the ether as signs, archetypes, and imagery, and translating it into holograms."[3] We are constantly communicating with all aspects of our Creator Matrix. We are just beginning to understand the power of this communication network and our significant role within it. Perhaps we will come to understand how we connect through our glycans to our information fields and our DNA networks. As we grow in consciousness and our DNA expands from two active strands to twelve or more, the consequences of this are beyond our comprehension at this point. I am convinced that instant manifestation and creating our reality will be the norm.

Co-creating and Manifesting: Using the "Oven of Grace"

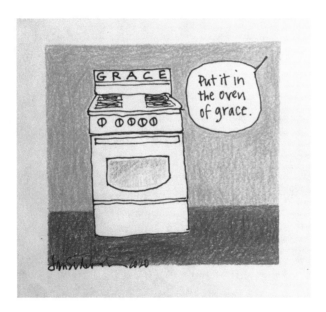

Each of us has our own unique journey of awakening. What will unify us as we awaken will be our integrated Creator Matrix and mastery of our creative abilities. Eventually, as we transform and make many changes, what seemed impossible to us will become possible. Mastering our Creator Matrix will seem effortless. As we learn to live multidimensionally in high-frequency wellness, we will be able to connect to all the elements in nature. These elements are fire, water, air, earth, and ether. As our Creator Matrix becomes more aligned, we will be able to connect to these elements and move or transform them with our thoughts.

In the past, the ancient practice of alchemy articulated these concepts and ignited people's imagination. Alchemists searched for ways to change matter. In particular, they tried to transmute common metals like lead and iron into silver or gold. They were motivated to do this as a way of curing disease and/or extending life.[4] For a long time, this seemed like impossible thinking. But, given what we now know, perhaps the idea that we can change the materialistic world directly is not so far-fetched. In many religions, there have been mystics and masters who seem to defy our common laws of physics. Walking on water? Changing water into wine? Demolecularization for time travel? Why not? The idea is based on the understanding that all matter contains a universal spiritual force, and science is proving this to be true.

Eventually, humanity will wake up to how powerfully our thoughts impact the materialistic world. If you think it and truly believe it, you will see changes in your life. A conscious Creator masters this ability. As we grow in consciousness, we will learn how to connect to and read the frequency of everything.

As we have learned, matter is made up of vibrating particles. If we can connect to the frequency of anything and everything, we can influence it. We can begin by connecting to the frequency of life force in nature. When we do so, we have the ability as Creators to move and transmute the elements. Eventually, we will become so good at this that we will do things that seem to go against the laws of nature (at least, as we understand them today). For example, if we were to connect to the frequency of the outer wall of a building, we could change our frequency to be in alignment with that wall; in this way, we could do what seems impossible, namely walk through that wall. However, in order to master such skills, we must have complete faith and no fear. We will manifest instantly when we have aligned our faith and beliefs completely with what we wish to manifest. Divine synchronicities will guide us, following our inner knowingness will become self-evident, and inner wisdom will direct our rightful action so this new power is not misused or misplaced.

A tool that I use when teaching my students to connect to the Universal Field is the "Oven of Grace." We all have this oven within us. It helps us to manifest intentionally and multidimensionally. Many of us know that, when cooking a dish, we need to prepare the food and place it in an oven for a certain period of time in order for it to manifest its form. We don't have to go into the oven to control it; in fact, if we open the oven door too soon, we may ruin the food. Our creative process works in much the same way. When we have an intention, we allow thought forms to gracefully drop into our "oven." We trust the universe to "cook" our desire and manifest it in its own perfect time. Learning not to control it is the secret. Complete trust is necessary. If our desire fails to manifest while in our oven, it is not the right path for our highest good at this moment in time. The old and familiar saying, "Be careful what you wish for," also applies to the Oven of Grace. Be conscious and aware of the intentions you place in your oven. In fact, be in love with what you put in your oven. Then, ensure that your container is big enough to handle such a manifestation. I encourage my clients and students to gracefully drop their goals and dreams into their oven and then let it cook. Much like heat emanates from the oven as we are cooking, our thought forms create a ripple of creation in the Universal Field. Knowing this, we can wait patiently for the manifestation to show up in its own divine time.

A New Beginning

Humankind is heading toward a new time, referred to by many as the Golden Age! We are ascending and awakening and ultimately remembering and reconnecting to who we really are: divine, conscious co-Creators and, in fact, consciousness itself. The basis of this is unconditional love. This love is eternal and, therefore, never dies. We simply change form as we evolve and experience ourselves anew, over and over again.

As we are all unique co-Creators, each of us will play our part in this time of transformation. Some, by their very nature and life purpose, are challenging old structures and helping to bring down the old paradigms, much like the proverbial sandcastle needs first to be destroyed before being rebuilt anew. At the same time, others are in the process of creating a New Earth.

What will the New Earth look like? I find this a difficult question since, each time I reflect on this and try to envision it, I realize that we can't know exactly because it hasn't been created yet. One thing is for certain: it will be vastly different to our current reality!

The biggest change will come from owning our power as Creators. We must realize that we, ourselves, are solely responsible for creating our lives. Each person must learn to take responsibility for themselves, and especially for their own well-being. Being well is also a frequency. Part of our learning is that everything you do with your body, mind, and spirit matrix is important. You must nurture it, love it, and care for it every day. Wellness, balance, and harmony will become the norm. As we ascend out of duality, complete wellness will become our baseline. Our light essence will shine brightly as we will have mastered the ability to hold high levels of light. In this book, we have learned the importance of both clearing and building the Creator Matrix. Our Creator Matrix is like a container; if it is clogged and full, we will be unable to completely utilize its true power. Once we learn to keep our container coherent, clear, and in perfect harmony, we will need for nothing as we will be integrated, whole, and open for the new.

As our consciousness evolves, we evolve, and we change. Imagine there are different stops and different routes we can take in our lives. You take care of yourself, feel great and get on the A Train one morning. Being in the flow, you meet your soulmate, and begin a life together. Or you don't take care of yourself, you're sick and tired in bed, you miss the A Train, and your life has a very different outcome, which becomes a different timeline. In essence, our timelines are directed by our conscious choices. This process of becoming never stops as we continue to evolve and increase our consciousness.

"Becoming" requires us to have the courage to create, digest, release, and integrate what our life experiences have brought us and how they have changed us. As we look at who we have become with love and acceptance, we can connect to a feeling of wholeness. As we ground the spiritual aspects of our higher self into our body from the Universal Field, we will integrate our Creator Matrix and step into our full potential. Some call this "being superhuman"; I believe that this is how we will create Heaven on Earth. Being the Creators that we are, we have a choice in how quickly we integrate these upgrades and make the necessary changes to embody this new superhuman status. This process of "becoming" will continue for eternity because we are eternal, and our consciousness is forever evolving.

Once fully aligned and well, our Creator Matrix will sparkle with crystalline energy in perfect universal geometry that will be expressed as perfect structure, sacred geometry. Structure is function, and we will master our Creator Matrix to manifest a world beyond our dreams. We will learn to manifest more quickly by being "other-focused" and connected to the collective heart consciousness. What used to appear like "magic" or seemed impossible will become our daily experience. Love and connection will continue to be the driving force that unites us as individual, and yet connected, Creators. Many have called this Unity Consciousness or Christ Consciousness; this state of being is the ultimate goal for humanity.

My wish for you is that you continue to grow in consciousness and continue to own and care for your Creator Matrix with love and joy. How will you allow transformation in your life? What will be the next steps on your journey? What is your mission with regard to the ascension and restoration of Planet Earth? None of us yet know the full scope of what is to come—but I know that, with the information in this book, you are now better prepared and aware to navigate it with love, grace, and ease.

I wish you a life filled with growth in consciousness, joy in your journey, unconditional love for yourself, and optimal wellness across all dimensions of your Creator Matrix.

Chapter Summary

- It is a powerful choice of transformation to decide not to suffer and not to judge, and to take full responsibility for creating our own life. This will help to create the new loving Earth we are all seeking.

- Where judgment is about "right" and "wrong" (often based in limiting beliefs), discernment is our ability to choose what we put our energy toward as Creators, and what we allow in our personal energy field and life story.

- As we grow in consciousness, we will choose safety over fear. We will learn to use our energetic field to transmute energy to feel safe even in uncertain circumstances.

- Spiritual awakening and raising our frequency will change our relationship with ourselves and—as a consequence—relationships with others. We will learn to discern which of our relationships are for a reason (to learn a lesson), a season (to serve our creative storylines at a moment in time), or a lifetime (true heart/soul connections).

- When we can forgive, we become free of distorted thought patterns, cut energy cords, and release the stored emotions; and we can transmute the darkness and only keep the lessons learned. Connecting to the frequency of gratitude for everything and everyone we encounter will shift our frequency instantly.

- When we learn to live from our hearts in a state of unconditional love and acceptance of all that is, we can move from a world of duality, conflict, and competition, and create a world of cooperation and coherence.

- We will become in complete alignment with our Creator Matrix. Each of us will step into our own sovereignty and hold higher and higher frequencies of light and love.

- In this new time, the definition of compassion is changing from feeling pity and concern, sympathy and empathy, and needing to interfere with other people's stories, into allowing other people their Creatorship and their stories, and only offering help when we are asked to do so.

- Through complete acceptance of any situation as it is, or whatever is showing up, feelings of resistance and fear can change into feelings of love. Humor, laughter, and joy can help tremendously to immediately change energy and raise the frequency.

- As we are awakening, our DNA is awakening, and we will gain more abilities and manifestation will become instant.

- As we grow in consciousness, we will learn how to connect to and read the frequency of everything, influencing the physical, materialistic world. We will be able to connect to the life force in nature and move and transmute the elements (fire, water, air, earth, and ether) with our thoughts.

- Divine synchronicities will guide us, following our inner knowingness will become self-evident, and inner wisdom will direct our rightful action.

- We can use our "Oven of Grace" to connect to the Universal Field, by making intentions and allowing thought forms to be gracefully dropped into our "oven." Complete trust in the process and not controlling it are the secrets for the universe to manifest it in its own perfect and divine time.

- Humankind is heading toward a new time and each of us will play our part in this transformation. The ultimate goal for humanity is the state of being which is called Unity Consciousness or Christ Consciousness.

Endnotes

Introduction

1.   Chávez, César. Address to the Commonwealth Club in San Francisco, Nov. 9, 1984. https://www.goodreads.com/quotes/47934-once-social-change-begins-it-cannot-be-reversed-you-cannot. Accessed Jan 2024.

Chapter Two

1.   Wagner, Paul. "This Theory Could Unify Consciousness, Matter, and Space." *Gaia*, July 2020. https://www.gaia.com/article/quantum-revolution-Einstein-aether-and-the-unified-field-theory. Accessed Jan 2024.

Chapter Three

1.   "Belief." Merriam-Webster.com Dictionary, Merriam-Webster, https://www.merriam-webster.com/dictionary/belief. Accessed Jan 2024.

2.   Mcleaod, Sue, PhD. "Freud's Theory of the Unconscious Mind." Simply Psychology, Oct 2023. https://www.simplypsychology.org/unconscious-mind.html. Accessed Jan 2024.

3.   "Personality." American Psychological Association (online). https://www.apa.org/topics/personality. Accessed Jan 2024.

4.   Almaas, A.H. *Keys to the Enneagram: How to Unlock the Highest Potential of Every Personality Type*. Shambhala, 2021.

5. Lapid-Bogda, Ginger, PhD. *Consulting with the Enneagram. Enneagram in Business*, 2015; pp 58-59, 91.

6. "The Nine Enneagram Type Descriptions." The Enneagram Institute (online). https://www.enneagraminstitute.com/type-descriptions. Accessed Jan 2024.

7. Lapid-Bogda, Ginger, PhD. *Bringing out the Best in Everyone You Coach.* McGraw Hill, 2009; p 26.

Chapter Four

1. "Key Concept #1: The Illness-Wellness Continuum." thewellspring.com. http://www.thewellspring.com/wellspring/introduction-to-wellness/357/key-concept-1-the-illnesswellness-continuum.cfm.html. Accessed Jan 2024.

2. "The Wellness Wheel." thewellspring.com. http://www.thewellspring.com/wellspring/introduction-to-wellness/364/the-wellness-wheel.cfm.html. Accessed Jan 2024.

3. "Stress." The Free Dictionary, Farlex, https://medical-dictionary.thefreedictionary.com/stress. Accessed Jan 2024.

4. "What Is Metabolic Syndrome?" www.heart.org/en/health-topics/metabolic-syndrome/about-metabolic-syndrome. Accessed Jan 2024.

5. Hannibal, Kara E., Bishop, Mark D. "Chronic Stress, Cortisol Dysfunction, and Pain: A Psychoneuroendocrine Rationale for Stress Management in Pain Rehabilitation." *Physical Therapy*, Dec 2014; 94:12; p 1816–1825. https://doi.org/10.2522/ptj.20130597. Accessed Jan 2024.

6. "Duality." Merriam-Webster.com Dictionary, Merriam-Webster, https://www.merriam-webster.com/dictionary/duality. Accessed Jan 2024.

7. "Stages of Change Model." Loma Linda School of Medicine (online). https://medicine.llu.edu/academics/resources/stages-change-model. Accessed Jan 2024.

Chapter Five

1. "Precession of the Equinoxes." *Encyclopedia Britannica*, March 2023. https://www.britannica.com/science/precession-of-the-equinoxes. Accessed Jan 2024.

2. Doody, D. "Basics of Spaceflight. Chapter 2: Reference Systems." *NASA* (online), https://science.nasa.gov/learn/basics-of-space-flight/chapter2-1. Accessed Jan 2024.

3. "Sunspots and Solar Flares." *NASA*, July 2021. https://spaceplace.nasa.gov/solar-activity/en/. Accessed Jan 2024.

4. "Sunspots and Solar Flares." *NASA*.

5. Alabdulgader, Abdullah, et al. "Long-Term Study of Heart Rate Variability Responses to Changes in the Solar and Geomagnetic Environment." *Nature News*, Nature Publishing Group, Feb 2018. https://www.nature.com/articles/s41598-018-20932-x. Accessed Jan 2024.

6. Kafatos, PhD, Menas C. et al. "Biofield Science: Current Physics Perspectives." *Global Advances in Health and Medicine* (online), Nov 2015; 4(Supplement): 24-34. DOI: 10.7453/gahmj.2015.011.suppl. Accessed Jan 2024.

7. Hurd, Sherrie. "What Is Schumann Resonance and How It Is Connected to Human Consciousness." *Learning Mind* (online), Jan 2021. https://www.learning-mind.com/schumann-resonance-human-consciousness/. Accessed Jan 2024.

8. Dispenza, Joe. "What Does the Spike in The Schumann Resonance Mean?" *Unlimited with Dr Joe Dispenza* (online), Feb 2017. https://drjoedispenza.com/blogs/dr-joes-blog/what-does-the-spike-in-the-schumann-resonance-mean. Accessed Jan 2024.

9. Loeffler, John. "What Is the Double-Slit Experiment, and Why Is It So Important?" *Interesting Engineering* (online), Feb 2022. https://interestingengineering.com/science/what-is-the-double-slit-experiment-and-why-is-it-so-important. Accessed Jan 2024.

10. "Akashic Records." *Academic Accelerator* (online). https://academic-accelerator.com/encyclopedia/akashic-records. Accessed Jan 2024.

11. Sohn, Emily. "Decoding the Neuroscience of Consciousness." *Nature* (online), July 2019. https://www.nature.com/articles/d41586-019-02207-1. Accessed Jan 2024.

12. McFadden, Johnjoe. "Integrating Information in the Brain's EM Field: The Cemi Field Theory of Consciousness." *Neuroscience of Consciousness*, 2020; Vol 1, niaa016. https://doi.org/10.1093/nc/niaa016. Accessed Jan 2024.

13. "Intuition–It's More than a Feeling." *Association for Psychological Science* (APS) (online), Apr 2016. https://www.psychologicalscience.org/news/minds-business/intuition-its-more-than-a-feeling.html. Accessed Jan 2024.

14. "Intuition—The Human Sixth Sense." *Yoga Digest*, Mar 2017. https://yogadigest.com/intuition-human-sixth-sense/.

15. Lufityanto, G; Donkin, C; Pearson, J. "Measuring Intuition: Nonconscious Emotional Information Boosts Decision Accuracy and Confidence." *Psychological Science*, May 2016; 27(5):622-34. DOI: 10.1177/0956797616629403.

16. Childre, D; Howard, M; Rozman, D, PhD; McCraty, R, Ph.D. *Heart Intelligence, Connecting with the Heart's Intuitive Guidance for Effective Choices and Solutions.* Waterside Productions, 2017.

Chapter Six

1. "Reconnective Healing & The Personal Reconnection." *The Reconnection* (online), Aug 2023. www.thereconnection.com/reconnective-healing-the-personal-reconnection/. Accessed Jan 2024.

2. "Quantum Mechanics." *Wikipedia*, Oct 2021. https://simple.wikipedia.org/wiki/Quantum_mechanics. Accessed Jan 2024.

3. Squires, G. Leslie. "Quantum mechanics." *Encyclopedia Britannica*, Dec 2023. https://www.britannica.com/science/quantum-mechanics-physics.

4. Sundermier, A. "99.9999999% Of Your Body Is Empty Space." *ScienceAlert* (online), Sep 2016. https://www.sciencealert.com/99-9999999-of-your-body-is-empty-space. Accessed Jan 2024.

5. "Electric Universe Theory." *The Electric Universe Theory* (online). https://www.electricuniverse.info.

6. Kafatos, PhD, Menas C. et al. "Biofield Science: Current Physics Perspectives." *Global Advances in Health and Medicine* (online), Nov 2015; 4 (supplement): 24-34. DOI: 10.7453/gahmj.2015.011.suppl. Accessed Jan 2024.

7. Kafatos, PhD, Menas C. et al.

8. "Plasma, Matter, and the Projection of Reality: Part 1." *Unlimited with Dr. Joe Dispenza*, July 2021. https://drjoedispenza.com/dr-joes-blog/plasma-matter-and-the-projection-of-reality-part-i. Accessed Jan 2024.

9. "Plasma, Matter, and the Projection of Reality: Part 1." *Unlimited with Dr. Joe Dispenza*, July 2021. https://drjoedispenza.com/dr-joes-blog/plasma-matter-and-the-projection-of-reality-part-i. Accessed Jan 2024.

10. McMahon, Mary. "What Is an Electromagnetic Field?" *All the Science* (online), Nov 2023. www.allthescience.org/what-is-an-electromagnetic-field.htm. Accessed Jan 2024.

11. Science of the Heart: Exploring the Role of the Heart in Human Performance. HeartMath Institute, 2015; Ch 6. https://www.heartmath.org/research/science-of-the-heart/energetic-communication/

12. "The Principle of Vibration [Tao]." *SuperPhysics* (online). https://www.superphysics.org/research/hermes/kybalion/chapter-09. Accessed Jan 2024.

13. Stone, Randolph. *Energy: The Vital Polarity in the Healing Art, Book 1.* R. Stone, 1957; p 20.

14. Hamlaoui, K. "The Human Body Frequency." ResearchGate, Mar 2020. https://www.researchgate.net/publication/340232697_The_human_body_frequency. Accessed Jan 2024.

15. "Hulda Clark." *Energy Medicine Research* (online). https://www.energy-medicine.org/hulda-clark.html. Accessed Jan 2024.

16. "The Frequency Generation." huldaclark.com. https://www.huldaclark.com/the-frequency-generation.pdf. Accessed Jan 2024.

17. "Hulda Clark." https://www.huldaclark.com. Accessed Jan 2024.

18. "Belief System." *Psychology Dictionary*, July 2015. https://psychology-dictionary.org/belief-system. Accessed Jan 2024.

19. "15 Quotes from Buddha to Help You Find Inner Peace." Power of Positivity (online), May 2023. www.powerofpositivity.com/quotes-from-buddha-inner-peace. Accessed Jan 2024.

20. "Neuroscience." *Oxford Learner's Dictionary*. https://www.oxford-learnersdictionaries.com/definition/english/neuroscience. Accessed Jan 2024.

21. Marks, J, MD. "Definition of Neuroplasticity." *RxList* (online), June 2021. www.rxlist.com/neuroplasticity/definition.htm. Accessed Jan 2024.

22. Thomas, S P, et al. "Anger and Cancer: An Analysis of the Linkages." *Cancer Nursing*, Oct 2000; 23(5):344-9. DOI: 10.1097/00002820-200010000-00003

23. Bailey, R. "The Limbic System of the Brain: The Amygdala, Hypothalamus, and Thalamus." *ThoughtCo* (online), Mar 2018. https://www.thoughtco.com/limbic-system-anatomy-373200. Accessed Jan 2024.

24. Pert, Candace B. *Molecules of Emotion: Why You Feel the Way You Feel.* Scribner, 2003.

25. *Summary of Candace B. Pert's Molecules of Emotion.* IDB Publishing, 2020.

26. Russo, A F, PhD. "Overview of Neuropeptides: Awakening the Senses?" *Headache*, May 2017; 57(Suppl 2): 37-46. DOI: 10.1111/head.13084

Chapter Seven

1. Navis, A R. "Epigenetic Landscape." *The Embryo Project Encyclopedia*, Oct 2007. https://embryo.asu.edu/pages/epigenetic-landscape. Accessed Jan 2024.

2. "Germany and the UK Collaborate to Train the next Generation of World-Leading Experts of Epigenetics in Single Cells." MRC Laboratory of Medical Sciences (LMS) (online), Mar 2019. https://lms.mrc.ac.uk/germany-and-the-uk-collaborate-to-train-the-next-generation-of-world-leading-experts-of-epigenetics-in-single-cells/.

3. Lipton, Bruce, PhD. "Brain versus Gonads." brucelipton.com, Feb 2012. www.brucelipton.com/brain-versus-gonads/. Accessed Jan 2024.

4. Lipton, Bruce, PhD. "Brain versus Gonads."

5. "You Can Change Your DNA." HeartMath Institute (online), July 2011. https://www.heartmath.org/articles-of-the-heart/personal-development/you-can-change-your-dna/. Accessed Jan 2024.

6. Ornish, Dean, et al. "Changes in Prostate Gene Expression in Men Undergoing an Intensive Nutrition and Lifestyle Intervention." *Proceedings of the National Academy of Sciences of the United States of America*, Jun 2008; 105(24): 8369–8374. DOI: 10.1073/pnas.0803080105.

7. Phillips, Theresa. "The Role of Methylation in Gene Expression." *Nature Education*, 2008; 1(1):116. https://www.nature.com/scitable/topicpage/the-role-of-methylation-in-gene-expression-1070/. Accessed Jan 2024.

8. "What Is Epigenetics?" Centers for Disease Control and Prevention (online), Aug 2022. https://www.cdc.gov/genomics/disease/epigenetics.htm. Accessed Jan 2024.

9. "What Is Noncoding DNA?" MedlinePlus (online). https://medlineplus.gov/genetics/understanding/basics/noncodingdna/. Accessed Jan 2024.

10. De Vogli, R, PhD. "Negative Aspects of Close Relationships and Heart Disease." Archives of Internal Medicine, 2007; 167(18):1951-1957. DOI:10.1001/archinte.167.18.1951.

11. *Science of the Heart: Exploring the Role of the Heart in Human Performance.* HeartMath Institute, 2015; Ch 6. https://www.heartmath.org/research/science-of-the-heart/energetic-communication/

12. "The Intention Experiment." Lynne McTaggart (online). https://lynnemctaggart.com/intention-experiments/the-intention-experiment. Accessed Jan 2024.

13. "Evidence." Lynne McTaggart (online). https://lynnemctaggart.com/intention-experiments/evidence/. Accessed Jan 2024.

14. "Evidence." Lynne McTaggart.

15. Gagliardi, E; Mondini, G. "DNA Modifications through Remote Intention: Semantic Scholar." *Neuroquantology,* Jan 2018; 16 (2018): 1-6. DOI:10.14704/nq.2018.16.1.1129.

16. Maier, M A; Dechamps, M C; Pflitsch, M. "Intentional Observer Effects on Quantum Randomness: A Bayesian Analysis Reveals Evidence Against Micro-Psychokinesis." *Frontiers in Psychology*, 2018; 9: 379. DOI: 10.3389/fpsyg.2018.00379.

17. McCraty, R; Tomasino, D. "Modulation of DNA Confirmation by Heart-Focused Intention." Semantic Scholar, 2003. https://www.semanticscholar.org/paper/MODULATION-OF-DNA-CONFORMATION-BY-HEART-FOCUSED-McCraty-Tomasino/94b61b4f33bfbac98deb0548a710641e73ef31f4. Accessed Jan 2024.

18. Dispenza, Joe. "Can You Change Your Brain by Thinking Differently?" *Unlimited with Dr Joe Dispenza,* June 2019. https://drjoedispenza.com/blogs/dr-joes-blog/can-you-change-your-brain-by-thinking-differently. Accessed Jan 2024.

Chapter Eight

1. Rath, S, et al. "Epigenetic Regulation of Inflammation: The Metabolomics Connection." *Seminars in Cell and Developmental Biology,* Feb 2024; 154(Pt C):355-363. DOI: 10.1016/j. semcdb.2022.09.008.

2. Vaucheret, H; Chupeau, Y. "Ingested Plant Mirnas Regulate Gene Expression in Animals." *Cell Research,* Jan 2012; 22:3-5. DOI: 10.1038/ cr.2011.164

3. Morello-Frosch, R, et al. "Environmental Chemicals in an Urban Population of Pregnant Women and Their Newborns from San Francisco." *Environmental Science and Technology,* 2016; 50, 22: 12464–12472. DOI: 10.1021/acs.est.6b03492.

4. Law, Larry. *There Is An Elephant in the Room: Exposing Hidden Truths in the Science of Health.* Angie's Option Inc GRM, 2017; p 179.

5. Hamishehkar, H, et al. "Vitamins, Are They Safe?" *Advanced Pharmaceutical Bulletin,* Dec 2016; 6(4): 467–477. DOI: 10.15171/ apb.2016.061.

6. Omenn, G S, et al. "Effects of a Combination of Beta Carotene and Vitamin A on Lung Cancer and Cardiovascular Disease." *New England Journal of Medicine,* May 1996; 334(18):1150-5. DOI: 10.1056/ NEJM199605023341802.

7. Davis, D R; Epp, M D; Riordan, H D. "Changes in USDA Food Composition Data for 43 Garden Crops, 1950 to 1999." *Journal of the American College of Nutrition,* Dec 2004; 23(6):669-82. DOI: 10.1080/07315724.2004.10719409.

8. "Controlling the Global Obesity Epidemic." World Health Organization (online). https://www.who.int/activities/controlling-the-global-obesity-epidemic. Accessed Jan 2024.

9. "Autotrophic Metabolism." *Encyclopedia Britannica* (online). https:// www.britannica.com/science/bacteria/Autotrophic-metabolism. Accessed Jan 2024.

10. Crampton, Linda. "Bacteria in the Large Intestine: Potential Effects on Health." youmemindbody.com, Sep 2022. https://youmemindbody. com/digestion/How-Do-Bacteria-in-the-Large-Intestine-Help-Us-Stay-Healthy. Accessed Jan 2024.

11. "20 Ways to Increase Your Vibrational Frequency." *Institute of Transformational Nutrition* (online), June 2018. https://transformationalnutrition.com/blog/science-of-nutrition/vibrational-frequency/. Accessed Jan 2024.

12. Honohan, J, et al. "Are Oreos Addictive? Nucleus Accumbens C-Fos Expression Is Correlated with Conditioned Place Preference to Cocaine, Morphine and High Fat/Sugar Food Consumption." Connecticut College Student Research, 2013. https://www.conncoll.edu/academics/internships-student-research/student-research-projects/are-oreos-addictive-nucleus-accumbens-c-fos-expression-is-correlated-with-conditioned-place-preference-to-cocaine-morphine-and-high-fatsugar-food-consumption.html. Accessed Jan 2024.

Chapter Nine

1. Contributor(s): National Research Council; Division on Earth and Life Studies; Board on Chemical Sciences and Technology; Board on Life Sciences; Committee on Assessing the Importance and Impact of Glycomics and Glycosciences. *Transforming Glycoscience: A Roadmap for the Future.* National Academies Press, Aug 2012.

2. Glycan Age. https://glycanage.com/.

3. Alavi, A; Axford, J S. "Sweet and Sour: The Impact of Sugars on Disease." *Rheumatology (Oxford)*, June 2008; 47(6):760-70. DOI: 0.1093/rheumatology/ken081.

4. Law, Larry. *There Is An Elephant in the Room: Exposing Hidden Truths in the Science of Health.* Angie's Option Inc GRM, 2017, p 113.

5. Defaus, S; Gupta, P; Andreu, D; Gutiérrez-Gallego, R. "Mammalian Protein Glycosylation – Structure Versus Function." *The Analyst*, June 2014; 139(12): 2944–2967. DOI: 10.1039/c3an02245e.

6. Gutiérrez-Gallego, R. "Glycans participate in multiple mechanisms of cellular regulation (illustration)." https://www.researchgate.net/figure/Glycans-participate-in-multiple-mechanisms-of-cellular-regulation-The-general-functions_fig6_261957572. Accessed Jan 2024.

7. Moreno-Gonzalez, I; Soto, C. "Misfolded protein aggregates: mechanisms, structures and potential for disease transmission." *Seminars in Cell & Developmental Biology*, May 2011; 22(5): 482–487. DOI: 10.1016/j.semcdb.2011.04.002

8. Alavi, A; Axford, J S. "Sweet and Sour: The Impact of Sugars on Disease." *Rheumatology (Oxford)*, June 2008; 47(6):760-70. DOI: 0.1093/rheumatology/ken081.

9. Schulze-Makuch, Dirk. "There Are More Viruses on Earth than There Are Stars in the Universe." *Air & Space Magazine*, Smithsonian Institution, Mar 2020. https://www.smithsonianmag.com/air-space-magazine/there-are-more-viruses-earth-there-are-stars-universe-180974433. Accessed Jan 2024.

10. Schulze-Makuch, Dirk.

11. Arney, Kat. "Viruses: Their Extraordinary Role in Shaping Human Evolution." BBC Science Focus (online), Aug 2020. https://www.sciencefocus.com/the-human-body/virus-human-evolution. Accessed Jan 2024.

12. Arney, Kat.

13. Spalding, K. L, et al. "Dynamics of hippocampal neurogenesis in adult humans." *Cell*, June 2013; 153(6):1219–1227. DOI:10.1016/j.cell.2013.05.002

14. Johns Hopkins University Press Office. "Sugar-Studded Protein Linked to Alzheimer's Disease." *Neuroscience News*, May 2022. https://neurosciencenews.com/glycan-alzheimer-20679/. Accessed Jan 2024.

15. Johns Hopkins University Press Office. "Sugar-Studded Protein Linked to Alzheimer's Disease."

16. Stancil, A N; Hicks, L H. "Glyconutrients and perception, cognition, and memory." *Perceptual and Motor Skills*, Feb 2009; 108(1): 259–270. DOI: 10.2466/PMS.108.1.259-270.

17. Han, Y S; Lee, J H et al. "Fucoidan protects mesenchymal stem cells against oxidative stress and enhances vascular regeneration in a murine hindlimb ischemia model." *International Journal of Cardiology*, Nov 2015; 198 (2015):187-195. DOI: 10.1016/j.ijcard.2015.06.070

18. Irhimeh, M R; Fitton, J H; Lowenthal, R M. "Fucoidan ingestion increases the expression of CXCR4 on human CD34+ cells." *Experimental Hematology*, June 2007; 35(6): 989–994. DOI: 10.1016/j.exphem.2007.02.009.

19. Espinosa-Marzal, R M, et al. "Sugars Communicate through Water: Oriented Glycans Induce Water Structuring." *Biophysical Journal*, June 2013; 104(12): 2686–2694. DOI: 10.1016/j.bpj.2013.05.017.

Chapter Ten

1.   Vocabulary.com Dictionary, s.v. "incarnate." https://www.vocabulary. com/dictionary/incarnate. Accessed Jan 2024.

2.   "Metaphysics." *Wikipedia*, Aug 2022. https://en.wikipedia.org/wiki/ Metaphysics. Accessed Jan 2024.

3.   "Mysticism." *Wikipedia*, June 2022. https://en.wikipedia.org/wiki/ Mysticism. Accessed Jan 2024.

4.   "Evolution: Definitions." Wordnik.com. https://www.wordnik.com/ words/evolution. Accessed Jan 2024.

5.   Mallonee, Laura. "Turns out Crystallized DNA Is Crazy Pretty." *Wired* (online), Aug. 2015. https://www.wired.com/2015/08/linden-gled-hill-crystalized-dna. Accessed Jan 2024.

6.   Lipton, Bruce PhD. "How Our Thoughts Control Our DNA." brucelipton.com, June 2014. https://www.brucelipton.com/how-our-thoughts-control-our-dna. Accessed Jan 2024.

7.   Poponin, V. "The DNA Phantom Effect: Direct Measurement of a New field in the Vacuum Substructure." Unpublished laboratory notes, 1995. Duplicating Experiments: Poponin, V; Gariaev, P. "Vacuum DNA Phantom Effect In Vitro and its Possible Rational Explanation." *Nanobiology*, 1995.

8.   Rein, G, PhD; McCraty, R, PhD. "Local and Non-Local Effects of Coherent Hart Frequencies on Confirmational Changes of DNA." 2001. https://www.semanticscholar.org/paper/LOCAL-AND-NON-LOCAL-EFFECTS-OF-COHERENT-HEART-ON-OF-McCraty/a0d9fca1c5cda01fcd2897fcc8a31f2836346af7. Accessed Jan 2024.

9.   SF, Anton. "Dr. Fritz Albert Popp: Biophotons." *Infopathy*. www.infopathy.com/en/posts/dr-fritz-albert-popp-biophotons. Accessed Jan 2024.

10.   "Biophoton Light." American Biophoton Association (online), americanbiophotonassociation.com/biophoton-light/. Accessed Jan 2024.

11.   "Biophotons: Humans Are 'Beings of Light.'" Premier Research Labs, Nov 2023. https://prlabs.com/blog/biophoton-fritz-albert-popp.html. Accessed Jan 2024.

Chapter Eleven

1. "12 Immutable Universal Laws." Laws of the Universe. https://lawsoftheuniverse.weebly.com/12-immutable-universal-laws.html. Accessed Jan 2024.

2. Ladd, Lorie. *The Divine Design*. Lorie Ladd LLC, Aug 2022.

3. Wheelock, Tobey. "Some Fundamental Ideas from the Law of One/ Ra Material." The Law of One, Feb 2020. https://www.lawofone.info/ synopsis.php. Accessed Jan 2024.

4. Sagan, Carl. "Cosmos - Carl Sagan - 4th Dimension." YouTube, Mar 2009. www.youtube.com/watch?v=UnURElCzGc0.

5. "Pierre Teilhard De Chardin." *Encyclopedia Britannica* (online). https:// www.britannica.com/biography/Pierre-Teilhard-de-Chardin. Accessed Jan 2024.

6. Grim, J; Tucker, M E. " Biography of Teilhard de Chardin." American Teilhard Association (online). https://teilharddechardin.org/ teilhard-de-chardin/biography-of-teilhard-de-chardin. Accessed Jan 2024.

Chapter Twelve

1. Sarkar, Donna. "20 Brilliant Quotes from Albert Einstein, the Theoretical Physicist Who Became World Famous." *Discover Magazine* (online), Mar 2023. https://www.discovermagazine.com/the-sciences/20-brilliant-quotes-from-albert-einstein-the-theoretical-physicist-who. Accessed Jan 2024.

2. "When Lorenz Discovered the Butterfly Effect." OpenMind BBVA (online), May 2015. https://www.bbvaopenmind.com/en/science/ leading-figures/when-lorenz-discovered-the-butterfly-effect. Accessed Jan 2024.

3. Kafatos, PhD, Menas C. et al. "Biofield Science: Current Physics Perspectives." *Global Advances in Health and Medicine* (online), Nov 2015; 4(Supplement): 24-34. DOI: 10.7453/gahmj.2015.011.suppl

4. Johnson, C; Green, B. "100 Years After the Flexner Report: Reflections on Its Influence on Chiropractic Education." *Journal of Chiropractic Education*. Fall 2010; 24(2): 145-152. DOI:10.7899/1042-5055-24.2.145.

5. Gøtzsche, P C. "Our prescription drugs kill us in large numbers." *Polskie Archiwum Medycyny Wewnetrznej*, 2014; 124(11): 628–634. DOI: 10.20452/pamw.2503.

6. Law, Larry. *There Is An Elephant in the Room: Exposing Hidden Truths in the Science of Health.* Angie's Option Inc GRM, 2017; p 59.

7. Levin, R, et al. "US Drinking Water Quality: Exposure Risk Profiles for Seven Legacy and Emerging Contaminants." *Journal of Exposure Science & Environmental Epidemiology*, Sep 2023. DOI: 10.1038/s41370-023-00597-z.

8. Fang, C, et al. "China's Improving Total Environmental Quality and Environment-Economy Coordination since 2000: Progress toward Sustainable Development Goals." *Journal of Cleaner Production*, Feb 2023; 387: 135915. DOI:10.1016/j.jclepro.2023.135915.

9. Yang, T, et al. "Effectiveness of Commercial and Homemade Washing Agents in Removing Pesticide Residues on and in Apples." *Journal of Agricultural and Food Chemistry*, 2017; 65 (44); 9744-9752. DOI: 10.1021/acs.jafc.7b03118.

10. "Amazing Ocean Cleanup Technology and Initiatives." Ecotourism World (online), April 2022. http://ecotourism-world.com/amazing-ocean-cleanup-technology-and-initiatives. Accessed Jan 2024.

11. Feinstein, D; Eden, D. "Six pillars of energy medicine: clinical strengths of a complementary paradigm." *Alternative Therapies in Health and Medicine*, Jan-Feb 2008; 14(1): 44–54.

12. Brand-New Online Retreat with Brandon Bays, courses.thejourney.com/the-journey-intensive/?orid=11716&opid=110. Accessed 6 Nov. 2023.

13. Ali, Mubashir. "The Day Science Begins to Study Non-Physical Phenomena, It Will Make More Progress in One Decade ..." Medium, Aug 2023. https://mubashirali786.medium.com/nikola-teslas-quote-on-non-physical-phenomena-c066db2c336. Accessed Jan 2024.

14. Lynn, Gail. "Energy Therapy from the Harmonic Egg® / Ellipse®." https://harmonicegg.com/energy-therapy. Accessed Jan 2024.

15. "The Blu Room®." Blu Room Wellness Center, https://bluroomwellnesscenter.com/what-blu-room/.

16. "What Is Eesystem?: Energy Enhancement System™." Energy Enhancement System (online), Jan 2022, https://www.eesystem.com/what-is-ee-system. Accessed Jan 2024.

17. Langdon, Larry. "What Is MedBed Technology?" SentientLight (online), Mar 2023. https://www.sentientlight.com/articles/ what-is-medbed-technology. Accessed Jan 2024.

18. "How Dr. Peter Goldman developed the Zone Technique." The Zone Technique (online). http://zoneschoolofhealing.com/zone-technique. Accessed Jan 2024.

19. Diesel, Norianna. "Intrinsic Data Field Technology." Norianna Diesel (online). https://www.norianna-diesel.com/quantum-scalar-energy. Accessed Jan 2024.

Chapter Thirteen

1. "Forgive/Forgiven - Aphiemi." Precept Austin (online), March 2023. https://www.preceptaustin.org/forgive-aphiemi-greek-word-study. Accessed Jan 2024. www.preceptaustin.org/forgive-aphiemi-greek-word-study. Accessed 6 Nov. 2023.

2. Vocabulary.com Dictionary, s.v. "coherence." https://www.vocabulary. com/dictionary/coherence. Accessed Jan 2024.

3. Gadbois, Linda. " DNA-the phantom effect, quantum hologram and the etheric body." MOJ Proteomics Bioinform, Jan 2018; 7(1): 9-10. DOI: 10.15406/mojpb.2018.07.00206.

4. "Alchemy." *Encyclopedia Britannica* (online). www.britannica.com/ science/chemistry/Alchemy. Accessed Jan 2024.

Acknowledgments

I extend this personal dedication to my ancestors (past and future) and most especially to those in my present, namely my large extended family (grandparents, aunts, uncles, cousins), and friends, all of whom have profoundly shaped and shared my life's journey. Your enduring spirits, unyielding support and love have woven a rich tapestry into my story, and for this I am profoundly grateful.

A special tribute goes to my husband, Frans. In our forty years of committed love, your steadfast support has been my guiding light. I also want to honor my children, Dr. Frans Jr., Kate and fiancé Floris-Jan, and Emma, who have all been my mirror and a constant source of my soul's growth, development, and inspiration.

I also dedicate this book to my parents, Robert (Bob) and Stephanie(†); my stepmother, Sally; my stepfather, Rod(†); my siblings, Christin, Jim, Paul, Robin, and Deborah, and their partners, Tom, David, Zahi, Vanessa, Kevin, Christopher, and Tiffany. I honor the next generation, the new children, all my American nieces and nephews: Bobby, Laura, Charlie, Franklin, Matt, Sam, George, Leo, Gus, Joe, Nicky, Phineas, Samantha, Dillon, and Lily.

A sincere dedication is offered to my parent's-in-laws, Frans Sr.(†) and Marianne, whose love and support have been constant and enduring, especially following my relocation to the Netherlands. This dedication further extends to my husband's siblings, Patricia, Alexander, Boudewijn, and Janneke, along with their partners, Douwe, Clarine, Eveline, Oya, and Marc, as well as all my European nephews and nieces: Kier, Mees, Alex Jr., Max, George, Boudy Jr., Frederique, fiance Alexander, Charlotte, Lucas, Melchior, Amadeo, partner Noa, Louis, Noepy, Rembrandt, Olympia, and Marc-Anthony.

***

Furthermore, I want to say a special thank you to the extraordinary souls who played pivotal roles on my journey and supported me to create this book.

Heartfelt appreciation extends to my sister, Deborah, for the priceless time and countless hours invested in thoughtful conversations about this project. Thank you for infusing your creativity and contributing beautiful and thought-provoking pictures that not only enhance the understanding but also inspire the reader.

Special thanks to my sister Robin, who generously helped with my professional picture, and to my brother Jim, who helped with the book launch.

A special acknowledgment is owed to Jeanneke, whose unwavering presence illuminated the path throughout the creation of both my course and this book. Her exceptional writing skills, infectious humor, and unconditional love have been a guiding light on this incredible journey.

Sincere gratitude to my friend and co-worker, Jeff, who generously lent his expertise from the project's inception, and who dedicated time to brainstorm and craft the initial draft with me.

Appreciation also finds a place for Karin, a steadfast pillar of support who stood by my side, offering invaluable assistance in organizing and researching the information.

A heartfelt thanks is reserved for Bryna, my publisher, who dedicated a year to restructuring and rewriting the material, transforming it into a well-organized framework that the world can truly appreciate.

Special appreciation goes to Eveline, my sister-in-law, whose guidance has been a constant source of strength, consistently helping me connect to my life's true purpose.

Appreciation extends to my daughter Kate and my friend Mylena for their generous contribution to our social media campaign, and for their assistance with the book launch.

I would also like to thank Larry Law, who has helped with the edits and a great inspiration as a teacher of the new sciences.

Lastly, profound gratitude to all my healers, therapists, teachers and guides who have helped me on my journey, particularly José Vergroesen(†), Dr. Lonsdorf, Dr. Levin, and Titia Licht.

Most especially, I want to thank the members of A Wellness Revolution, a community of lightworkers and colleagues. Your steadfast support over the years has played an instrumental role in the mission to bring about vital education and change needed for healing and the co-creation of a new world filled with light, love, and fulfillment.

About the Author

Cathleen Beerkens is a dedicated health professional with a diverse background in nursing and a passion for holistic wellness and healing. Holding a BS degree in Health Education from the University of Maryland and a BSN from Georgetown University, Cathleen embarked on her nursing career at Georgetown University Medical Center in Washington, D.C.. Over twelve years, she gained invaluable experience in various medical settings, including the emergency room, medical/surgical ward, high-risk labor and delivery units, and as a teaching assistant at the Georgetown University Nursing School.

In 1996, Cathleen's journey led her to Amsterdam, the Netherlands, where she and her husband raised their three children. Intrigued by integrative medicine, she delved into different forms of healing beyond conventional Western medicine. Recognizing the limitations of her medical background, Cathleen studied and received certifications in ancient and contemporary healing practices, such as Polarity Healing, reflexology, and Reconnective Healing. She spent many years researching and helping people heal on all levels of body, mind and spirit. Her pursuit of knowledge culminated in her graduation from the Institute

381

of Integrative Nutrition in 2017 as a certified health coach.

Driven by a desire to share her insights with the world, Cathleen founded A Wellness Revolution in 2018, an organization dedicated to training and certifying health and wellness coaches globally. The curriculum focuses on cellular well-being, with an emphasis on epigenetics, neuroscience, quantum physics, glycoscience, and a holistic vision of health and wellness. A Wellness Revolution aims to address contemporary healthcare challenges by providing a deeper understanding of self-care through cutting-edge scientific perspectives.

Cathleen's holistic healing and coaching practice, developed over many years, has empowered her to witness remarkable transformations in individuals. Her students, comprising doctors, therapists, practitioners, nurses, entrepreneurs, lifestyle coaches, and those seeking a conscious health-driven life, benefit from her expertise. Cathleen believes in the profound impact of conscious living on one's path and future self. Her genuine love for helping people improve and regain their health is evident in the daily miracles she witnesses. Through A Wellness Revolution, Cathleen continues to be a catalyst for positive change in the global landscape of health and wellness.

Learn more about Cathleen's work and find a board-certified health and wellness coach at www.AWellnessRevolution.com.

About the Illustrator

Deborah Caiola is an artist and educator working between Los Angeles and Philadelphia. Winner of the Leeway Foundation's Transformation Award, Caiola works passionately to champion feminist ideals through her art. In her practice of painting, illustration, printmaking, and digital art, she attempts to create with presence and to allow the medium and the experience of making to direct her work so that the product is a combination of planning and improvisation. Paramount to Caiola's work are the ideas of connectedness and compassion, believing that art can be a guide and advocate for these and many other joyful human pursuits. Learn more at www.DeborahCaiola.com.

About the Publisher

Founded in 2021 by Bryna Haynes, WorldChangers Media is a boutique publishing company focused on "Ideas for Impact." We know that great books change lives, topple outdated paradigms, and build movements. Our commitment is to deliver superior-quality transformational nonfiction by, and for, the next generation of thought leaders.

Ready to write and publish your thought leadership book with us? Learn more at www.WorldChangers.Media.

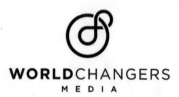